Praise for *Wellmania*

'At last! A funny, well-written work of first-person gonzo reportage concerning all the health and serenity treatments you've ever been too feeble personally to undertake. Think of this book as an entertaining semi-colonic.'
—Annabel Crabb

'Brigid Delaney is the queen of calamity and a fearless, sane guide into the bizarre heart of our modern obsessions. This will make you groan in horror as much as it'll make you laugh out loud.'
—Benjamin Law

'A bloody entertaining read that leaves you wondering whether you want to do yoga and meditation or get mindlessly drunk and despair at the state of the world. Basically I wish that I'd written it.' —Judith Lucy

'Her search is earnest, and she's game for just about anything, but Delaney is also unflinching in her examination of the darker side of the wellness industry'
—Jenni Kauppi, *Books+Publishing*

'[An] entertaining romp through the "wellness industrial complex"'
—Fiona Capp, *The Sydney Morning Herald*

'Delaney is funny and unashamedly honest, capturing the nuance of emotion we all feel when trying to be more "well".'
—*Fashion Journal*

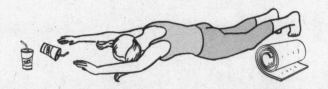

WELLMANIA

MISADVENTURES
IN THE SEARCH FOR WELLNESS

BRIGID DELANEY

CORONET

Originally published by Nero in 2017,
an imprint of Schwartz Books Pty Ltd

22–24 Northumberland Street
Collingwood VIC 3066
enquiries@blackincbooks.com
www.nerobooks.com

First published in Great Britain in 2023 by Coronet
An Imprint of Hodder & Stoughton
An Hachette UK company

This paperback edition published in 2023

1

A CIP catalogue record for this title is available from the British Library

Paperback ISBN 9781399718271
eBook ISBN 9781399718257

Printed and bound in Great Britain by Clays Ltd, Elocraf S.p.A.

Hodder & Stoughton policy is to use papers that are natural, renewable and
recyclable products and made from wood grown in sustainable forests.
The logging and manufacturing processes are expected to conform to the environmental regulations of the country of origin.

Hodder & Stoughton Ltd
Carmelite House
50 Victoria Embankment
London EC4Y 0DZ

www.hodder.co.uk

CONTENTS

For Tim & Bonnie – two friends I admire
who live well, but also live good.
And for Frankie – who's just beginning.

PREFACE

When I wrote *Wellmania* in 2015 and 2016, the wellness industry seemed to be an unstoppable beast. Influencers, Instagram, wellness tourism, hot yoga, controversial detoxes, paleo, colonics, bone broth, raw food, superfoods, silent meditation retreats, no-sugar diets, ten-minute workouts, smoothie bowls, mindfulness apps, infrared saunas, sound baths, ayahuasca journeys, injectables for the masses ... there were so many ways you could improve yourself.

But then, of course, it all stopped. In 2020 we shut our doors and stayed inside. We couldn't get to the yoga retreat in Thailand, or even to the yoga class up the road.

But, in a way, wellness became more important than ever. We were all trying to stay well and not get the virus. Protecting society's health became the central organising principle of government. The wellness trends that had loomed so large only a few years before now seemed to belong to a different era.

This book, *Wellmania,* was examining those trends, but also reaching for something larger. Beyond all the commerce, the busyness, the money, the hacks and the products – were there things that could lead to us feeling *better*?

And was there a way of doing wellness that wasn't tied to the market, or having money, or mobility, or a fully operational hot bod?

Could wellness actually mean feeling creative, connected, in community and engaged in meaningful work?

And if that's what wellness meant to me, how did I go about getting it? How did we *all* go about getting it?

The journey in this book was my search for wellness after I turned forty in a messy, chaotic fashion. I was living in Bushwick, New York, in a sublet of a sublet of a sublet. I don't think it was a space designed to be lived in. I slept on a makeshift bunk, dangerously close to exposed piping that may or may not have been slowly gassing the apartment. We were being evicted. I was earning scraps of money doing food and travel stories on the ten best cocktails in Manhattan rooftop bars, or the five best po' boys in New Orleans. But winter was coming, I was about to be homeless and money was low. I went out the night before my birthday – a blur of drinks, dive bars and stumbling around unfamiliar streets. The next day, the day of my birthday, I was the most hungover I'd ever been. I felt unwell – very unwell. I knew something had to change; *I could not go on like this*! Maybe the wellness industry had the perfect product to turn my ship around?

I returned to Australia on the promise of just one magazine assignment. I was asked to write about a radical detox during which I might just hit all my wellness goals in one wild ride. The detox plan was to not eat any food for fourteen days, then restrict myself to one piece of chicken, an egg or some cucumber for a total of 101 days. After that, not only would I be skinny, I would be well.

What happened with that detox is described in often horrific detail in the first section of *Wellmania*. The second section deals with fitness and the body – in particular, all things yoga. The last section looks at spirituality.

Did I find the wellness I so desperately needed? Let's just say I'll never do another detox again.

One person who loved the book was Australian writer Benjamin Law. He was approached by the TV production company Fremantle with an open brief: If he could make any book into a TV show, what would it be? He chose *Wellmania*. For him, the bigger themes of connection and community resonated and, living in Sydney, he saw the comic potential of all these wellness trends that we were so invested in – at least until the next trend came along.

In the writers' room for *Wellmania*, everyone had different ideas of what wellness meant, but we shared universal experiences too. We'd all worried about our own health at some point, and had seen people we love get sick and sometimes die. We were all, at some time or another, conscious that our bodies were not conforming to the wellness ideal, or that our minds were not as settled and as calm as the meditation apps told us they should be.

We realised there was a very human and very relatable story in striving for wellness, not quite getting there, but picking yourself up and trying again.

And even more relatable? Realising that once you achieved your goal, the things that you were actually looking for – community, connection, creativity, wholeness, acceptance – were yours for the taking all along.

Brigid Delaney
Byron Bay, June 2022

BEFORE

I n the last days of my thirties, I was living in a warehouse in
Bushwick, Brooklyn. It had never really felt like a home.
Strange and beautiful murals by the Iranian artists Icy and
Sot ran five metres up the building, a former storage facility.
The walls were flimsy, and painted X's in the stairwell marked
demolition or some future work to be undertaken. We had a loft
bedroom in which guests slept centimetres from exposed pipes
leaking something that wasn't poisonous, but wasn't pleasant. We
always kept the windows open, even when it was cold.

I was sub-sub-subletting it from an Australian photographer
who had moved to Kabul, but no one seemed to know who was
on the lease. Mail came for at least a dozen different people with
exotic names; Germans, Russians, Koreans and Welsh people had
all lived here. We knew them by their uncollected bills.

Winter was coming. I was finishing edits on a novel and had
settled into a nice routine. Breakfast was a toasted poppyseed
bagel with hummus and a large, strong latte over the paper edition of the *New York Times* at a cafe that played old Smiths songs.
There were happy-hour margaritas with friends in Manhattan,
dinners at bistros around Brooklyn – farm-to-fork stuff, with
an emphasis on the produce of Vermont (in particular, bacon).

My yoga studio was near home, at the back of a dive bar. You did a class for twelve dollars and got a free pint of beer. When the deadline for my novel drew near, I took prescription-only diet pills and worked with a furious focus for eighteen hours a day.

On my birthday, I pretended to be an Asian friend to get access to her private members club in the East Village. My friends and I were meant to go on to a Daft Punk tribute band, then have supper at a place up in Harlem, but instead sat around until after midnight drinking Negronis and Old Fashioneds from heavy-bottomed crystal glassware – the sort that in Agatha Christie novels were used as murder weapons. Later – a speakeasy filled with really young people, the season's first snow, cold legs, the frightening sight of my face in the bathroom mirror (the assistant at Sephora had gone all goth with my eye make-up), my friends going to another bar to buy some molly – and me drunk, disorientated, walking somewhere in Chelsea, then in a cab, arguing with the driver about the best way to get home. Him getting upset, telling me over and over to 'stop cussing'.

The next night I went to my real birthday party, with friends who made me cake. I sat very still, sipping tea, feeling disconnected, unwell. I was terribly hungover.

My twenties and teens had been years of living wildly. I'd had a debauched thirtieth in Barcelona that was meant to be goodbye to all that. Yet my thirties had been reckless and exhilarating in a way I hadn't expected. It felt like I was a ball and someone was playing pinball really hard with me. I was shooting all over the place, the board lighting up and the music playing.

What did I want my forties to look like? Not this. The carnival was over. Yet, yet, the fun I had … My friends were the same.

Children had slowed some of them down, but the things that were meant to happen – the brakes applied, the early bedtimes, the slippers and the hot chocolate – had never eventuated.

After my birthday we got evicted from the warehouse. It was the first time I had just walked out of an apartment with all the stuff still in it. When I slid the keys under the door, there were still jumbo tubs of mayonnaise in the fridge.

I headed south. In Jakarta a couple of years before, I had met a Texan guy. He ran a boutique hotel near the diplomatic district and the first time we met we'd stayed up all night on the roof of the hotel, the pool shimmering and the call to prayer sounding at 4am from the mosque below. That first conversation, mostly about books and writing, lasted until the sun came up. I wondered if this could be love. He was the biggest hedonist I'd met. He was now back in Texas and the prospect of seeing him again filled me with excitement, and a smattering of fear. He'd be picking me up from the airport in a red Cadillac.

But first, Atlanta. I went in face-first, eating Americana – baked sweet potato covered in marshmallows and coated in Splenda, with hunks of cola-basted baked turkey for Thanksgiving. Then the bus to Savannah: drinking in the streets, Spanish moss, pretty graveyards and this place called Angel's Barbecue, where I first tasted, and adored, proper southern cooking.

Then a week in New Orleans for a travel story: a sign at the airport saying this was the number-one city for liver transplants, a band that looked and sounded like The Cat Empire playing for hours in a backstreet of the French Quarter under shifting shafts of sunlight, mint juleps, martinis, shots of bourbon – appropriately – on Bourbon Street, jazz bars, gumbo. Reviewing a restaurant called

Mother whose side portions of mac and cheese spread across enormous dinner plates.

Then, finally, Austin with my Texan friend, who had grown a beard and put on 12 kilos since Jakarta. Restaurants, brunches, Tex-Mex, red wine, chess in front of an open fire at the W, live music, beer, house parties, cocaine, melted cheese dip and corn chips, football games, women in cowboy boots cracking on to my Texan, me feeling sick with jealousy, no sleep, meeting a woman who had 'blown every rocker in Austin' and was obsessed with the novels of Tim Winton. Nachos, enchiladas on hot plates, hot dogs on paper plates, tequila at brunch, rib joints, burger bars, piano bars, martini bars, dive bars. Starting to feel unwell all the time, my body protesting, actually aching at the excesses.

On my flight back to New York an elderly woman collapsed. They laid her out in the aisle and the plane dipped into LaGuardia and slid down the runway as fast as I've seen a plane land. She was fitted with an oxygen mask and taken out of the plane on a gurney. Her friends filed out behind her, alarmingly unconcerned. They were Texans coming to New York for Christmas shopping. The sick woman was a portent. I felt it. I also returned from the South feeling about 100 years old. Every part of me was tired.

Back in New York, it was freezing. There was snow on the footpath, and the pine scent of freshly cut Christmas trees was in the air. I was not quite homeless. I had agreed to cat-sit in a building on the Upper East Side, for a friend of a friend. This woman lived in a room without any windows with a cat she had found in a dumpster. The cat's name was George Costanza.

The room used to be a storage cupboard. That's why it had no windows. I was shocked that a cat could live in such a small space, let alone a human being. I quickly felt depressed in the airless bed-sit with the scared, unhappy cat. Without a proper kitchen, I ate all my meals at a nearby diner: eggs always coming with something called hash, bad coffee in bottomless cups.

Sometimes I'd have dinner at my friend Brendan's house. He was trying to quit sugar. We ate pasta, drank vodka tonics and smoked outside. He talked of the withdrawals – irritability and headaches, cravings and crankiness – like sugar was a drug. His street ended with a sudden drop to an embankment leading to the long, thin Riverside Park that ran all the way down to West 72nd Street and, beyond the park, to the Hudson River. We stood out in the dark, facing the water. But I was thinking of a different body of water – one I always returned to.

Bondi. December. The way the sun made the cliffs golden in the late afternoon. The daily swims, the briny air and the strong coffees. I missed it so much. It was a place that exuded a vital sort of health, a honey-baked splendour. I didn't know if beautiful people moved there, or if you became beautiful by living there, submitting to the rhythm of the place: running on the beach, surfing, laps of Icebergs, all that yoga, all that meditation, all that warming sun.

I yearned to feel healthy again. I didn't feel sick, but I did feel sub-optimum, lethargic. Aching joints on the inside, a coat of grease on the outside, spotty and paunchy with bloodshot eyes. My clothes were tight. My mood was low. 'Don't put me on Facebook!' I had to say more than once, as friends took my photo. I needed to lose about 20 kilograms to get back into a healthy weight range. I needed, basically, to reset my body and my life. I yearned for a different way – a more virtuous way. I wanted to be clean.

Just at this time, a curious opportunity landed in my inbox. It was a magazine assignment. Would I be interested in writing a first-person account of a controversial fast that lasts for 101 days? Malcolm Turnbull, the man who would in 2015 become Australia's prime minister, had done it. His weight loss was so dramatic, people initially speculated he had cancer.

Fasting – according to Google – means not eating.

The assignment would entail returning to Australia and, for the first month, attending a clinic every day for massage and acupuncture, followed by a daily weigh-in. For the first fourteen days I would be allowed *no* food, instead subsisting on foul-smelling herbs taken three times a day.

It was almost too difficult to contemplate, and yet too enticing to ignore. It didn't just promise weight loss. It also promised to detox me, to cleanse my organs and restore them to their optimal functioning. I would look younger, metabolise food faster (when I was back to eating), think clearer, even smell nicer. Sure, it would be like signing up for the New York Marathon without ever having run for the bus, but I thought the fast might 'shock' me into good health. Wellness entrepreneurs such as Gwyneth Paltrow endorsed fasting, and if it's good enough for Gwyneth ...

I contacted my old housemate in Bondi. Yes – my room was available. It was close to the fasting clinic.

I booked a ticket back to Australia and prepared to return home to detoxify myself.

It wasn't just a detox I was after. A quick fix wouldn't suffice. I needed to give my system a hard reset. I was not only flabby but also plagued by mood swings and low-level discontent. I was sick of this pattern of swinging from health kick to hangover and back again. A detox would be a great initial purging of my sins, but I also needed to get toned and then work on creating some semblance of equilibrium – an inner life that held me steady, that provided a deep well of wisdom, and was some sort of ballast for when times got tough.

If I had these boxes ticked – if I could be clean, lean and serene – then I would be living my best possible life. Wouldn't I?

The search for these things led deep into the heart of the vast complex of companies and individuals making money from all those millions of us in search of a better body, a more balanced inner life, and clean and high-functioning organs: the wellness industry.

The wellness industry is a global behemoth, worth around US$3.4 trillion annually, making it nearly three times larger than the $1 trillion pharmaceutical industry. It includes vitamins, beauty and anti-ageing, fitness, mind/body, weight loss and healthy eating, wellness tourism, workplace wellness and spas.

I had been dipping in and out of this mega-industry for around a decade before I started on my hard reset. The road to wellness has been my own personal stations of the cross. My job as a travel journalist meant I was lucky enough to try different, sometimes wacky, wellness products, often in far-flung places. I've done meditation, yoga, drinking opium with Brahmin priests, retreats in Benedictine monasteries, volunteer work in Japanese Zen Buddhist temples, being lathered in oil and basted like a barramundi at an Ayurvedic compound in the jungle of Sri Lanka, raw food diets and a program of colonics in the Philippines after my blood work revealed the degraded profile of a lifelong meat eater. I've fought against my Irish potato genes in an effort to become leaner, signing up to hot yoga challenges and strenuous multi-day hikes.

There have been lots of stumbles and falls, acts of kindness, revelations, insights and moments of beauty along the way. I've learnt what works for me and what is a waste of time and money.

I am not naturally lean, clean or serene. I love feeling good, but I also love a good time. To hit my pleasure zones I will often use the shortcuts of alcohol, unhealthy food and lolling about with a book (Fitbit recording a grand total of forty-eight steps for the day). I've tried all these wellness experiences because I am genuinely curious about whether any of this stuff works.

Will they give us a lithe body, a long lifespan, a sense of meaning and purpose? Will they give us calm and certainty and happiness in a world where so few old certainties and beliefs remain? Will we be better people afterwards, stronger and more successful? And will any of this stuff actually make us happier? Or is it just some giant capitalist project designed to take all our money but never properly sate us? From a distance, the wellness industry can seem like a spinning wheel for caged mice: on and on we run, focused on our own individualistic goals, looking straight ahead, running, running, running.

But we rely on the industry because things are so out of whack. Many of us in the West – those privileged enough to have time and a disposable income – are living in times of high decadence. We swing from excess to self-imposed deprivation with dizzying speed and frequency. There's the Christmas holiday binge followed by the February detox; the weekend of alcohol and cocaine followed by a week of sweating out the toxins in hot yoga; the mindset meditation apps that you can use when you need a quick break from multi-tasking.

What I ask in this book is not just what the wellness industry offers – the deeper question is *why?* Why do we strive so deeply to be clean, lean and serene at this particular moment in time? What does the pursuit of these goals say about us? What is missing from our lives that leads us to seek spirituality in a yoga class, or community on a retreat, or purification through a diet?

This is the true story of one woman's adventures in the search for wellness, warts and all. It's the story of my expensive – and at times somewhat dangerous – voyage into a complicated and sprawling constellation of industries and products, some ancient, some new, all responding to or feeding on the craziness and insecurities of the modern world. And it's the story of all the genuinely useful stuff I've learnt along the way.

CLEAN

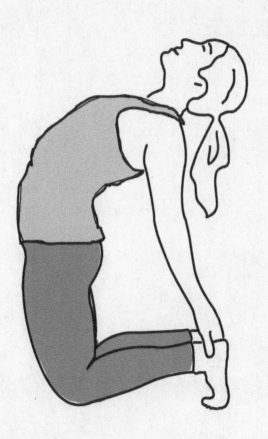

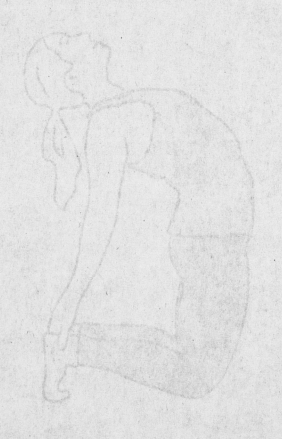

When I return home from America, the sensation I carry around in my body is an almost ever-present discomfort. I'm not feeling *sick* sick (apart from the jet lag: that heavy, weird feeling of your body arriving somewhere while another part of you – your soul, perhaps – is still travelling), but I'm not feeling *well* well. It's that discomfort many of us have. The discomfort of abundance. The discomfort of people who have too much, who do not need to move too far or too hard to get food, the discomfort of always feeling a little bit bloated and off, the discomfort of the desk-bound worker, bent and curved like a well-fed snake around the computer screen and office chair for eight, nine, ten hours a day. This is the discomfort of someone who can fit in a yoga class on the weekend or a walk to the shops, but tends to clock around 6000 or fewer steps a day. The discomfort of a person who drives to the supermarket, eats out a few times a week, once in a while will lose her shit on bourbons and Cokes, but mostly likes one or two glasses of wine a night. This is the discomfort of a person who has a lot on her mind and worries about the future, her work, her family, waking sometimes at 4am and having a hard time getting back to sleep. This is the discomfort of a person for whom exhaustion – or at least a low-level version, with its minor aches and pains, a bit of brain fog and forgetting names, the *hmpruff* sound made when bending to put on her shoes – is the new normal.

I have all that. My body feels like it has a tenant on a long-term lease trashing the place a bit. Not enough to get them evicted – not yet – but those tenants were not taking good care of the structure.

'I have a plan,' I tell my body. 'You may not like it. It's pretty dramatic, but hear me out. The plan is to kick out this bad tenant and do a major reno. It's going to be painful. There's going to be some demolition work – the foundations are going to be ruptured and rebuilt.'

'Hmmm …' says my body, a bit nervously. 'What are you going to do?'

'I'm going to starve you for as long as we both can stand it.'

Detoxes are controversial. It used to be that the word 'detox' was used to describe a medical procedure to wean addicts off drugs and alcohol. It was done in a treatment centre, under medical and psychiatric supervision. People detoxed if they had life-threatening addictions. It was a hair-raising, hang-on-to-your-hat sort of ride. People *died*.

Yet somehow the term 'detox' has entered the mainstream, uncoupled from its original meaning and co-opted by the wellness industry. There's detox tea, detox shampoo, detox oils, detox energy drinks, detox powders, detox juices, detox salads, detox books, detox apps and detox holidays. Detox programs available over the counter at pharmacies or on the internet promise to detoxify specific organs – or the whole body – and alleviate a range of symptoms. A happy side effect is weight loss – although many programs would not be so gauche as to say that on the box.

'Let's be clear,' says Edzard Ernst, emeritus professor of complementary medicine at Exeter University in an article in the *Guardian*. 'There are two types of detox: one is respectable and the other isn't.' The respectable one, he says, is the medical treatment of people with life-threatening drug addictions. 'The other is the word being hijacked by entrepreneurs, quacks and charlatans to sell a bogus treatment that allegedly detoxifies your body of toxins you're supposed to have accumulated.'

If toxins did build up in a way your body couldn't excrete, the professor says, you'd likely be dead or in need of serious medical intervention. 'The healthy body has kidneys, a liver, skin, even lungs that are detoxifying as we speak. There is no known way – certainly not through detox treatments – to make something that works perfectly well in a healthy body work better.' So basically, if you have internal organs, you're detoxing.

But what is a 'toxin'? Is it just a word that encompasses all our regrets?

The word derives from Greek and is defined by *Dorland's Medical Dictionary* as 'a poisonous substance produced within living cells or organisms' that can be capable of causing disease when absorbed by the body's tissues. It can be something that enters the body (like lead or pesticide), it can be found in drugs and alcohol, and it can also be poison found in nature such as a bee sting or snake bite.

But the word 'toxin', as thrown around in the wellness world, has come to have a fairly elastic meaning. It's toxins that make us feel sluggish and toxins that result in disease. It is too many toxins that rob us of our vigour and strip us of our health. Toxins are to blame for many of our modern maladies – the things that make us feel slightly off but not downright sick: the tiredness and exhaustion, the trouble sleeping, the bloating and constipation, joint pain and stiffness, the greasy pallor, the fat around our middles that won't go away (despite all the Pilates classes, all the stomach crunches), the dull hair, the weak nails, the colds and flus we pick up so easily at every change of season, the moodiness, the irritability, the low-level depression, the spikes of anxiety that wake us in the night. It's the word we reach for in January with our bodies weak from partying, the slightly sweaty-sour taste of last night's champagne still in our mouths, a receipt for a burger we don't remember buying at 2am, eaten in the Uber we don't remember ordering ... In contemplating all of this we utter the words that signal our edge, our limit, our end point, our surrender: 'I really need to detox.'

I really need to detox.

And we mean it, we really do.

Despite the faddishness of detoxing, fasting itself (or severe calorie restriction) has been around as long as humans have. We're evolved for it, due to the long periods between food faced by early hunter-gatherer man. When abundance – or at least supply – was established, fasting was co-opted for religious, moral and health purposes. Jesus fasted, as did Buddha and Gandhi.

Pre–Vatican II Catholic theology teaches that our mortal, impure bodies spend an unspecified time in the fires of Purgatory, where we undergo purification and healing. We need to undergo temporal punishment, according to the Roman Catechism, in order to cleanse ourselves from sin and start healing. All the major religions have incorporated some element of fasting into their catechism and calendars. Jews have Yom Kippur (the Day of Atonement). Muslims fast during Ramadan. Many Christians fast on Ash Wednesday and Good Friday, and on Fridays during Lent. Hindus fast on festival days.

Hunger is deeply linked to spirituality: fasting is seen by religion as a path to purity and enlightenment. It brings us closer to God. In being empty we are able to fully receive.

In 65AD, the Roman Stoic philosopher, statesman and dramatist Seneca advised his friend Lucilius: 'Set apart certain days on which you shall withdraw from your business and make yourself at home with the scantiest fare. Establish business relations with poverty.' Fasting loosened attachments to comfort and material possessions:

> Endure all this for three or four days at a time, sometimes
> for more, so that it may be a test of yourself instead of
> a mere hobby. Then, I assure you, my dear Lucilius, you
> will leap for joy when filled with a pennyworth of food,
> and you will understand that a man's peace of mind does
> not depend upon Fortune; for, even when angry she
> grants enough for our needs.

Socrates, Plato, Aristotle, Hippocrates, Pythagoras and Galen all advised short fasts to cleanse the mind and the body. 'Instead of employing medicines, fast a day,' advised Plutarch, the Greek biographer. Centuries later, Mark Twain agreed: 'A little starvation can really do more for the average sick man than can the best medicines and the best doctors ... starvation has been my cold and fever doctor for fifteen years, and has accomplished a cure in all instances.' A travel journalist I know recommends fasting for jet lag.

Yet the science surrounding fasting is minimal. I wonder: is the lack of science due to the fact that fasting is free and cannot be monetised or patented? After all, there is no need to take a pill and no need to spend any money. No drug company in the world has manufactured something that mimics the effects of fasting. The basic act of not eating is uncommodifiable. What we pay for is people to make us hold the line – people, as I was to find out, such as Dr Liu.

The detox I had signed up for was meant to last 101 days. The brochure promised that if I did it correctly, if I followed it to the letter, the program would restore my organs to their optimum working order, and I would live until I was 101 years old, disease free. But the regimen is not for the faint-hearted. It started with *no food* for fourteen days, before moving on to small amounts of solids: half a cucumber on the first day, 50 grams of poached chicken the next (think the size of three fingers), then an egg on the third day, then back to the cucumber. Repeat the cycle for the next sixty days. Black tea and water were permitted. The Chinese medicine, a mixture of herbs, was to be taken orally, three times daily. The herbs give you around 250 calories a day. So, although I might feel as if I was fasting (I was to eat nothing), Dr Liu has argued it's not to be called a 'fast' – it's to be called a detox, because of these calories taken in liquid form.

The night before I start the detox, I go out. It's one of those wild, hot Sydney nights where your table in the hotel beer garden swells and shrinks with people. Imagine a time-lapse video: we are three, then we are six, then we are fifteen, then we are twenty-five, then we are eleven, then we are six, then we are four;

cigarettes and empty glasses; bowls of chips; ice melting too quickly in the bucket, the wine bottles swimming and bobbing in a warming world.

Everyone is home for the summer. I am with Erik, Nick, Patrick and Joel. We are at the hotel, then we're at an artist's studio drinking whiskey and sitting on tins of paint, then we're at Oporto on Broadway and it's 3am and a man at the next table slides off his chair and sinks to the ground like his heart has just stopped.

Booze and parties still have their allure, but the allure is full of complications. I question whether I should be in Oporto at 3am; I stare at the man on the ground, thinking slightly dispassionately, slightly freaked out, that the difference between him and me is probably only one more drink. We are both here at 3am, tearing through the burgers like animals.

Yet earlier in the night, on the eve of my fast, I thought with a sureness that seemed so true and right: *I could never give this up. I don't want to give it up*. I love this kind of night – a group that is just right, made up of people I love, and who love each other, who have history with each other: brilliant, witty, each a star that is forever circling around others in our constellation.

It would be great, it would be so *great*, if only I could leave the party at 10pm, when it's in full swing. Instead it's just one more pub, just one more drink, yes to the cigarettes, yes to the shots at the bar, yes to the dram of whiskey, yes to the next place. I can never stop before the party stops.

Outside Oporto, waiting for an Uber, the sirens and swaying groups and taxis streaming past, I try to put some distance between me and the slumped man. Every atom of him is not every atom of me, for tomorrow things are going to change. I will be detoxing. And the detox will be a sort of moral excoriation, self-flagellation, a redress, a ferocious kind of back-burning that will run across the organs I'd abused. I'll be scorching something in order for it to grow again, refreshed and renewed. And at the end I would emerge – clean.

**

What I should have done is tail off gradually.

I should have cut down on caffeine a week – or ideally two – before such an extreme detox. The same with alcohol, meat, sugar, fast food and large portions. Smaller portions would have shrunk my stomach a bit. A detox doctor I meet later in Thailand tells me he puts all fasters on a no-protein, no-dairy, plant-based restrictive diet in the two weeks before they arrive, so the shock on their system when they stop eating is not so great.

Easing my body into the no-food thing would have helped it adjust. Instead I was going to feel like a plane suddenly dropping from 6000 feet to the runway. The landing was going to be rough. But I cling to my pleasures for as long as I can. In an echo of those more primitive detox clinics – the ones for the addicts – I turn up at the clinic with a hangover and a large, strong takeaway latte, determined to take my drugs of choice with me as close to the threshold as we are allowed to go.

The clinic is on level four, on the way to nowhere. You do not go to this part of the mall by accident – you go because you have an appointment, because you need something about your body fixed. Run by a Chinese medicine practitioner, Dr Shuquan Liu (his surname eerily prescient of where I would be spending much of my time in the later stages of the detox), the clinic is next to a botox place and looks blank and anodyne. Around it hangs the odour of wet and decaying branches, which I would later learn came from the Chinese herbs being prepared in a back room. The shopfront could be selling anything, or nothing. In a strange way, it is doing both. People are forking out thousands of dollars in order not to eat (it costs around $2000 a week). We are paying for an absence to be enforced.

At the clinic's front desk is a receptionist and a glass cabinet. In the cabinet are identical boxes filled with liquid herbs, waiting for collection. Each box is decorated with Chinese calligraphy and has a person's name on it. I discreetly try to read the names – my fellow fasters, doyennes of deprivation, soulmates in starvation. Maybe a celebrity is also doing the detox?

I am incredibly nervous. I have been anxious about the detox for weeks now and have thought about it almost constantly: what would it actually *feel like* to stop eating? Can I handle it? I've had a few dry runs of not eating for a day or so – but using super-strong prescription-only diet pills to stop the hunger. My relationship with food has been quite uncomplicated. I eat what I want, when I want. I share the Hannah Horvath (of *Girls*) view of dieting, which is that there is too much going on in life to devote time and mental space to 'food issues'.

Besides, my job as a travel writer often requires me to eat rich, beautiful food in some of the best restaurants around the world. One assignment had me travel to Bologna and eat twelve differ-ent bowls of bolognaise over two days. Pig livers and spinal cords, mashed eye mixed with blood and spice, pasta as light as hair – all washed down with Modena red. On a recent trip to Georgetown in Penang we ate – in *one day* – nasi goreng for breakfast, elevenses of elderberry pop and curry puffs in a marquee in the Malaysian jungle, a ten-course degustation for lunch at a new French-inspired, all-white-interior restaurant, high tea of scones and cakes at the jewel of the colonial Pacific – the Eastern & Oriental Hotel, canapés and champagne at an art gallery, a multi-course Chinese banquet for dinner, then supper at a nightclub where you could snack on Malaysian hawker cuisine. In one day. How on earth will I find the willpower to not eat for fourteen days (not a scrap, not a crumb, not a morsel) and then another eighty-six on a highly restricted diet? The only way I can imagine lasting that long without food is if I am put into an induced coma.

Mainly I am worried about any physical pain or discomfort that might arise from continual hunger. I also worry that I may die.

The receptionist sits me down and hands me a copy of *Harper's Bazaar* while I wait to see Dr Liu. In the magazine is an article by a journalist who has done the detox. She writes: 'Word-of-mouth converts grimaced about this mysterious, vile-smelling concoction you had to drink three times a day, adding it was the best thing they'd ever done. They warned me it was torture and required willpower because of the no-food factor. But I had to know more.'

I also have to know more. I wonder if I too will become a 'convert', 'grimacing' while swallowing the medicine.

I have read other things about the detox. It first came to prominence when the now Prime Minister Malcolm Turnbull and his wife, Lucy, did it. 'I must say that I found the fast extremely informative because it made me realise I am in control of my own body and can control my appetite. It is a very good insight,' Turnbull told the *Global Mail*. When Turnbull appeared in public after a break of several weeks, he looked dramatically different. People thought he had cancer. Since then he has kept the 14-kilogram weight loss off, but not publicly discussed the fast.

It isn't just Turnbull. There are other famous fasters, including members of Sydney's business elite: Aussie Home Loans founder John Symond (20 kilograms), PR supremo Max Markson and game-show host Larry Emdur (10 kilograms). It is a detox for a certain high-achieving class of Sydney men – power lunchers with a paunch.

Reading Rear Window in the *Australian Financial Review* or the Media Diary in the *Australian* you would see snippets of someone's incredible weight loss. Was it gastric banding? Was it lipo? No, it was Doctor Liu.

Dr Liu told the *Daily Mail*: 'Everybody should be at optimum health but many people have poor levels ... Food can't process because organs aren't working and they put on weight, they can't think straight, they are tired. We fill the gap between current health levels and maximum health levels.'

In response to Turnbull's rapid weight loss, warnings were issued about extreme fasting. The Australian Medical Association's vice president, Dr Geoffrey Dobb, told Seven News that starvation and herbal tea were not the answer to losing weight. 'Any rapid weight loss can be followed by a rebound if people are unable to sustain the program they have entered into,' he said. 'It's up to the individuals, but one would hope that people like Malcolm Turnbull use their influence responsibly.' The *Harper's Bazaar* writer white-knuckles it through the detox, although she has a few close calls. She must flee a black-tie banquet to avoid tempting platters of food. Starving, she returns to her hotel room and – in a scenario I will come to know well – looks at pictures of dessert on Instagram. But ultimately deprivation wins over desire and soon the weight is dropping off. She writes: 'When my personal trainer catches wind of what I've done he's furious. This goes against everything health professionals tell you, but I feel amazing.'

I don't have a furious personal trainer (instead I have a cautious and circumspect editor) but everyone is disapproving, intrigued and freaked out when I tell them I am not eating for two weeks and thereafter only permitted a small 'meal' of cucumber or an egg each day. My friend Erik applauds my move into this niche: a gonzo journalist for the wellness industry, a Breatharian version of Hunter S. Thompson. But many friends think what I am doing is unsafe. I've gone to my GP for advice – a sensible, lovely English guy who just shrugs and says, 'Keep an eye on how you feel, come and see me if it gets weird.' Then as a coda – and in an echo of Seneca – he mentions if anything, fasting will serve as a sort of moral instruction. 'So many people in the world go hungry and we have so much. You'll get to appreciate the true value of food, and what happens when it becomes scarce.'

He takes my blood pressure, which is at its usual hysterically high reading, and fills out a script for a new batch of pills to keep it down. He also prescribes statins for high cholesterol. I am too young to be taking these drugs.

When we have our first consultation, Dr Liu tells me that if I stick to his program, my blood pressure and cholesterol will lower dramatically and I'll be able to go off the medication. In fact, this is the one piece of science that has been proven time and time again with fasting – it's great for reducing hypertension.

'Come and see me when the fast is over and we'll see if anything has changed for you,' says my GP.

✳

At the counter of the detox clinic a man – late forties, corporate type, with a largish stomach and a well-fed – but not *fat* – face is negotiating with the receptionist. His issue is when to start – you see, he has this important dinner on, and he is going on holidays, then there is this crucial meeting, the sort of meeting you can't do on an empty stomach. His body tells a story of success without discipline, cutting a lavish figure under an expensive suit, the receptacle of good dinners and corporate lunches, too much time spent at a desk or at the pointy end of the plane. Coffee in the morning to wind him up. Booze in the evening to wind him down. He probably had the warning from his doctor, the same one I got – high blood pressure, crazy cholesterol, the tarot cards turning over, forewarning a heart attack.

But he is not looking into his future – he is looking at his diary and it is full of stuff. How can you detox when you have an important dinner coming up, or your own birthday party? Detoxing is what doesn't happen when life gets in the way. There is never going to be a good time to start.

My timing is okay. In fact it is probably ideal. I have no life to interrupt. I returned from New York a week ago with no job and no money. Undertaking a detox makes sense not only from a work and (possibly) a health perspective but also financially. Even if I wanted to eat, I can't afford it. I'm flat broke. My credit cards are maxed out. And there is no money in the future – no cheque coming my way, no job to start, no rich relative who is just hanging on.

As Seneca counselled Lucilius, a fast helps you 'establish business relations with poverty'.

January is just a bunch of blank pages in my diary. New Year's Eve I would spend alone – babysitting an infant. I've pulled up at a strange, silent junction in my life. There are a million interesting things behind me – and probably a million yet to come – but the present is a curious blank, non-time. Take a number and sit in the waiting room.

Not eating would be a further excursion into this non-time non-zone. The thought comes, the one I have been trying to keep at bay: forget my physical health, this could be very bad for my mental health. How much of a crutch is food, giving me structure and something to look forward to, providing me comfort?

Adrift in a sea of time, untethered from meals – can I cope with that?

Dr Liu calls me in. He is a Chinese man of neat and dapper appearance in his middle years but whose precise age I cannot guess. He is also very slim. At certain angles, with his hair slicked back, he appears to gleam. Behind the reception area is a long series of rooms set up with massage tables and cabinets for acupuncture needles and scales. Chinese people in white coats move between the rooms.

Dr Liu briefly explains the process I am about to undertake: during the first stage, lasting for about a month, the organs will cleanse and release toxins. Then stage two, also lasting for a month, is organ repair and recovery, while stages three and four are organ maintenance and balance. His manner is terse and watchful, yet also benevolent. He has a knowingness about him, like he has seen it all before and what is going to happen to you is okay.

Some of the claims made in his literature are a little wild – for example, if you stick to his program you will live until you are 101 years old. This is quite unappealing. I like the idea of living until my mid-nineties but anything beyond that seems excessive, and since I am the only person I know who is doing the fast I would enter my hundreds friendless, my more toxic friends having died long ago. Dr Liu also promises that if you complete the whole detox your body will maintain its new, good optimum health (and your new weight) for the rest of your life – which I am also sceptical about. What if you go straight back to fast food, degustations and boozing? The fast – even though it is extreme – sounds like a form of cheating if you can eat whatever you want for *the rest of your life*.

Yet his appointment book is full to bursting. He has five clinics across Sydney, Melbourne and Brisbane. Surely there is something here that works? In the brochure the clinic sends you before you start, your fears are pre-empted: 'It is important to trust both Dr Liu and what is a tried and test [sic] program with thousands of advocates. There will be moments of doubt and weakness but by finishing the journey and remaining mentally strong there are significant long term health benefits.'

The first step is assessing my general health. Dr Liu checks my pulse and observes my tongue, eyes and skin, before gauging how much oxygen is getting to my organs. I lie on my stomach as he swiftly heats up glass cups and puts them on my back. I know this is called cupping but have never experienced it before. There's a sort of strange, suction-y sensation on my skin as the cups are set down. He leaves the room and I can feel them pulling at my skin, like he put the nozzle of an almost-broken vacuum cleaner on my back. When he takes them off, Dr Liu shows me my bare back in a mirror. Gross. I look bruised, or like I've had a terrible spray tan.

'You are highly toxic,' says Dr Liu. 'These marks show that the oxygen is not reaching your organs.'

'What? What does that mean?' I ask, alarmed.

Apparently there is a lot of fat around my organs, preventing them from breathing properly. My fat is sort of crushing them.

The way Dr Liu describes it, this isn't the roll of fat on my stomach – this is fat *in* my body that is crowding my liver, kidneys and spleen. Thin people have this fat as well. Invisible fat. Invisible but deadly. Exercise won't shift it – not the fanciest gym, not the best personal trainer, says Dr Liu. Only a deep detox will work. If I follow his program, and clean my body from the inside out, eventually my organs will be able to breathe and function properly again. According to Dr Liu's promotional materials, 'The key factor in how much weight you will lose is the measure of fat around the stomach area. On average you will expect to trim 5 to 10 centimetres from your waist and 5 to 8 kilograms of weight in the first fourteen days.' This will 'improve both your immune system and general metabolism. By default your body will adjust to an ideal short and long term weight and body shape for a healthier, longer life.'

For the majority of the clinic's fasters, it really is all about the weight, when all is said and done. The program says it's about organ function, but weight – shedding it, dropping it, burning it, losing it – is the endgame. The number on the scales is your measure of success or failure – and in the curiously empty, strange and suspended zone that is your life while you are on the detox, anchorless in a world without mates or meals, it's the number on the scales that is the main motivation.

Of course weight will be lost. You're not eating.

But the no-food thing is not negotiable. In its own way, that very clear boundary means that the diet should be easier. You can't eat anything. So you eat nothing. Milder detoxes that involve elimination – no wheat, sugar, meat, dairy, alcohol or caffeine – can be easy to cheat on or at least renegotiate with yourself. This cake uses agave, which is not real sugar, so I'll just eat that, or this smoothie only uses a dollop of yoghurt – which won't really hurt – so I'll order that. When you are forbidden to eat anything, *everything* is cheating. And if you cheat, there is a feeling – a very strong feeling – that somehow Dr Liu will know. He emits a sort of spooky vibe, like he is there with you, in your home, as you negotiate with yourself whether to eat an almond.

But all this is ahead. Right now there is just fear and anticipation. Excitement, even. And there are the scales. There's no need to be scared – you may never weigh this much again!

Dr Liu watches impassively as I strip off to my underwear and step on those electronic scales that weigh you to the precise decimal point. I had been very careful not to weigh myself in America. I was in a beautiful northern-hemisphere magical thinking – winter when it should have been summer, night when it should have been day; I was eating like a thin person with the metabolism of a teenager but actually swelling up like a balloon. Now it was time to wake up from the magical thinking.

Woah. Okay. I'm awake now. That number is kinda large. Maybe it was the latte? The *large* latte.

But no matter – it has begun. I am to return to the clinic every day for weigh-in, massage and acupuncture – and the collection of more boxes of herbs. The daily treatment, according to Dr

Liu's materials, is designed to help your body release built-up toxins and fat more quickly and easily. 'Without daily treatment,' the brochure says ominously, 'you are unlikely to cope with the 101 Wellbeing Program.'

Wellness blogs frame the detox experience differently from my fears. It is not a hardship to be endured; rather I am giving my body a lovely holiday in which my organs and digestive system can just lie around the proverbial swimming pool and relax, order some nachos and put it on room service. Our bodies work hard: hours and hours a day digesting, breaking down, redistributing, burning, storing and expelling food and drink, pharmaceuticals, skincare and street pollution, fire retardants on sofas, etc. You are essentially an eating and shitting machine (or as the rock group TISM would have it, 'You eat, you shit, you die'). When you're not forcing it to enact this endless loop of digestion, your body can get around to doing other things – chores it has put off because it's been too busy. This is the cleaning bit that is so desirable these days. This cleaning and these chores might include repairing old wounds, cleaning out dead or diseased tissue and using these cells for fuel, pulling out toxins from tissues – like old medications or recreational drugs you had *years* ago – and processing them, repairing muscle damage, cleaning up scar tissue, expelling the excess mucus that hangs around in your body, protecting cells, removing all the old bits of meat and gristle that have been stuck to your colon wall for decades and draining you of all the excess fluid inside of you, being useless.

Jared Six, an artist who blogs about clean living and fasting, subscribes to this belief. He writes:

> The best analogy that I can use to describe fasting is to imagine that a grocery store closed for a week but all of the employees still showed up to work as usual that week ... Every inch of the floor could be cleaned and polished, all of the walls could be re-painted, all of the old electrical wiring could be stripped out and replaced with faster and more energy efficient wiring that would eventually save the store a lot of money in the long run, and when the week was over it would look like a brand new store on the inside and they could have a 'grand re-opening'.

A few years ago in the Philippines, chasing a clean body, I'd had my blood tested and they said the platelets showed the undesirable profile of a lifelong meat eater. To cleanse me, they quickly put me on a raw, vegan diet, and I spent the rest of the week eating shaved zucchini trying to pass itself off as pasta.

And it wasn't just meat. I was also an occasional smoker, regular drinker and a person who has tried Valium, LSD, hash, ecstasy, MDMA, cocaine, speed and marijuana. My store – to use Jared Six's analogy – was like one of those two-dollar shops with a storekeeper who was also a bit of a hoarder. There was cheap plastic crap from China clogging up the aisles, stuff was piled to the ceiling, and there were things shoved to the back with dust and dirt

all over them that no one had looked at for years. The *clean-up* –
such as it was – would be gruelling.

*

After I am weighed, Dr Liu gives me his mobile number and tells
me to contact him at any time during the program if I have questions or concerns. The receptionist hands me the boxes of herbs,
which have been made up especially for me – like a prescription.
It is all the food I need for the next two weeks. They are heavy –
so heavy that I need to make three trips on the bus to bring them
all home. I am to drink the herbs, which have been liquefied and
placed in individual sachets (like large packets of soy sauce), three
times a day.

When it's time for dinner, I drop the contents of a sachet in a
saucepan of hot water. Apparently they are more palatable heated
up. I probably should be more concerned that I am putting something in my body whose ingredients are unknown. Instead I focus
on the odour. It's cloying and medicinal, and smells like I've wandered deep into a woodland where an animal has died. Then the
taste ... imagine swigging from a flat beer the morning after a
party and discovering that there are ten cigarette butts floating
in the bottom. It is rank. But Dr Liu has assured me the herbs will
contain all the nutrients I need to get through the next fourteen
days without dying.

*

Researching fasting, I find old blogs from people who live in northern
California, in the woods, and haven't eaten for like ... ever. Scrolling
down long, long pages of sans serif fonts and late-1990s HTML is

both encouraging and alarming. Some of the blogs have pictures that look like conceptual art, but on closer inspection are the contents of very full, very messy toilet bowls. They have advice on DIY enemas and recipes for fast-breaking vegetable broth. They explain their shit to you in loving detail – its shapes, texture and odours.

Then I find a fascinating article in *Harper's* from 2012. It asks and tries to answer questions that keep on coming up for me – particularly in weeks two and beyond of the detox. Does fasting or detoxing have a healing mechanism, just like sleep? Is abstaining from food the path to vigour? And can you reverse some aspects of the ageing process through fasting and detoxing?

I am intrigued about what could happen to my body, apart from weight loss. There is a lot of mystery around it. How, for example, does detoxing affect metabolism long term? Dr Liu said little to clarify what is actually going on inside my body when I am starving it.

I find other first-person accounts of long detoxes and these read like wild, primitive experiments that are on the frontier of something, the way early researchers recorded their experiences with LSD. We don't know *why* this is happening to our bodies, or *how* – but this is *what* is happening. Candace Chua on her wellness blog and the late David Rakoff on *This American Life* (as well as Steve Hendricks in *Harper's*) went before me and detailed, imprecisely, lyrically, with wonder and bewilderment – what happened to their bodies, minds, relationships, work and emotions while they fasted for long periods of time.

Any results were of course impressionistic – not scientific. As it is here with me.

Day one of any diet and you're gung-ho and ready to go. I'm no exception. I plan to stay inside (*hide* inside) all day so I will not encounter any food out there in the wild. It is December in Bondi – party time in a hedonistic place. Icy plunges into the sea off the rocks at Ben Buckler, the sun warming the grass, the sandstone glowing the colour of buttery chardonnay, the hot white sand and smell of oil and sunscreen and perfume, the heat and bare bodies, salty skin, barbecues and cold beers as the sun goes down ...

It seems an affront to nature to stay inside. I can see the ocean from my window – deep blue, vital and shimmering. Breakfast is the herbs, of course. I pierce the packet with a knife, sending the warm brown liquid shooting onto my chest – like lancing a particularly fetid boil. I drink the herbs in the manner of a tequila shot. It becomes apparent I will always need to have a chaser of water handy to wash the taste away. I like the action of shooting the herbs, how the motion of my arm, with my head tipped back and a chaser at my elbow, carries echoes from a more debauched recent past.

The hunger I thought would appear on that first day doesn't. I am too waterlogged to feel hungry. In addition to the herbs I am drinking black tea with a bit of honey, and a load of water. I sort of slosh around the house in a restless and agitated state, waiting for the hunger pangs to hit.

I have only one thing to give the day – and all the days – shape: the visit to Bondi Junction to the clinic, where I am given traditional Chinese medicine treatment and weighed. Before I start the program, I am excited by the idea of a daily massage. It gives the whole enterprise a sort of day-spa, muzak, scented-oil indulgence. But I quickly discover this is not the case. The detox massage feels like being roughed up for your phone and wallet on a dark side street. The clinic workers pull at my legs and stomach, they press and they pinch, they knead me like a lump of dough and they stick their fingers deep into my stomach – presumably jiggling around my internal organs, as if loosening the jackets of fat around them. I come to dread the stomach massage even more than the needles.

After the rough massage, fifteen to twenty needles are applied to my bruised stomach and head, around the temples and in my hair. I then rest for a bit on one of the massage tables. After the needles are removed, I am weighed. Then it's home to drink my herbs, consume lots of water and rest. The next day, repeat, ad finitum.

So what's going on in my body in the early stages of the detox?

On the first day, six to twenty-four hours after beginning the detox (known as the post-absorptive phase) insulin levels start to fall. Glycogen breaks down and releases glucose for energy and these glycogen stores last for roughly twenty-four hours. Then gluconeogenesis (literally meaning 'making new glucose') occurs in the next twenty-four hours to two days. This is when the liver manufactures new glucose from amino acids. Glucose levels fall but stay within the normal range – providing you are not diabetic. This is the body using the last of its sugar supplies before it switches into ketosis – the fat-burning mode beloved by body builders, anorexics and paleo devotees.

On day two I discover I have lost a kilogram already – an even, satisfying one kilogram. 'It's working!' I say excitedly to the receptionist. The neatness of the number bodes well. My friends – who are sceptical of my detox – aren't so impressed. 'It's just water,' they say of the weight loss. 'You're probably pissing like a donkey.'

On day three I lose almost two kilograms – so that is almost three kilograms in three days. Is it still water?

It's good that progress on the scales is swift because week one without food is passing slowly, like a sickness or fever has taken hold. For the first couple of days I am restless, vaguely depressed and anxious. The jitters, muscle aches and intense headaches I put down to caffeine withdrawal. I'd been on three lattes a day and hadn't tapered off. Everything is heavy; I can feel the energy leeching out of me, as if it were physical matter escaping my body. Small movements such as filling up the saucepan with water feel strangely laborious, like I have been pumped full of lead or injected with some sort of tranquilliser. Outside my window, the sun is too strong – that bright Sydney light, making everything both too stark and too washed-out all at once. I lower the shades.

Yet, despite my lethargy, for the first few nights I can't sleep, jacked up on whatever is in the herbs. I feel speedy – but maybe it's the hunger. It's ferocious, and my only respite from thinking about food is when I go to sleep. Even then my empty belly wakes me at odd times: 12:30am, 4am, 5:23am.

In *One Day in the Life of Ivan Denisovich* Aleksandr Solzhenitsyn writes, 'The belly is an ungrateful wretch, it never remembers past favors, it always wants more tomorrow.' And more now. It wants more *now*. Yet I am also aware how staged this all is – I'm not Ivan Denisovich starving in a labour camp, with no way of knowing if or when the hunger will end, if it will end with – and be the cause of – my death. I can stop at any time. It is resisting food and temptation, not genuine scarcity, that I face. I may as well be sitting on the floor of a larder. I am surrounded by food.

✳✳

Detoxing for two weeks would be the most difficult thing I've done – but also the most interesting. Not only do you get to know your body in a different, fascinating and grotesque way, but the central place food and drink takes in our society is sharply illuminated when you take yourself out of the game. For a start, not eating removes you from a large segment of the economy. Suddenly there's all this stuff you can't buy: coffees, breakfast, lunch and dinners, drinks (in bars and bottle shops, coconut water, Coke or Gatorade from the servo), groceries, snacks. A whole world of restaurants and cafes becomes forbidden. I take fifty dollars out of the ATM on the first Friday of my new no-food life and it is still in my wallet on Monday. This has never happened before. It becomes startlingly apparent how much time, money and energy I spend procuring, preparing and eating food.

When I stop eating, suddenly huge amounts of time are freed up, long stretches of it punctuated by nothing. Time to spend thinking – about food. Humans have contemplated the potential of this absence from time to time: what if we were liberated from the drudgery of having to cook and clean up after ourselves? What if we lived in a post-food society? A post-food society could also be a post-feminist society – since most of the food-prep work traditionally falls on women. Think of the other things that could be achieved! All the projects, all the inventions, all the innovations, all the conversations, all the work and all the play.

Rob Rhinehart, a Silicon Valley nerd, tried it – living off packets of powered protein and supplements. He saved so much time, he said, he got so much work done. This was the way of the future. Become more productive, stop preparing and eating food – just buy his powdered product (called Soylent). It's now a multi-million-dollar business – and a 'disruptor' in our food-production cycle.

So what do I do with all this newly freed-up time?

Paradoxically, I find that while I have so many more hours in the day to do stuff, I am either too weak or too vulnerable to leave the house. On the street, I might encounter food. At one point I go out to get some more tea bags and end up walking blocks out of my way, following someone carrying a delicious-smelling box of pizza.

I try not to look at anyone eating, or stop and stare at any food outlets as I go up Bondi Road on my way home, but, oh man, it is hard. Food is all I can think about. I gravitate towards greasy spoons – the burger joints where only the most hungover unperson would cross the threshold, where the man behind the counter is handling a chemical sausage full of pink dye with his bare, tattoo-knuckled hands ... I just stand at the counter and watch, like a creep.

At home, in my room, depleted of energy, the only thing I do with any gusto is google 'cleanse', 'detox' and 'fasting', desperate to find people out there who are going through the same thing. All I discover is a patchwork of anecdotes on blogs, a lot of pseudo-science, strange theories and very little in the way of rigorous scientific research. There are – unsurprisingly – few of us that are eating nothing but herbs. The 5:2 diet is popular at the time, but the 0:7 diet is for outliers. Fasting is a political act, for the religious, the mentally and terminally ill or for sects such as Breatharians, who claim to live on air alone.

Most people in the forums on the internet are on juice cleanses that only last for a few days. Gwyneth Paltrow, with her much-maligned 'cleanse program' (people say it is too harsh, but compared with what I'm doing, it is a total walk in the park – there is some broth, some vegetables), is a solace and a spirit guide during this time.

The Queen of Clean – what would GP do? I ask myself later in that first week, lanced and bruised by the needles, swollen with sleep, disturbed by strange dreams – standing in the fridge light at 1am. I am staring at the olives. I am staring at the olives. I am staring so hard at the olives, but keeping my fists in a ball, so they can't reach in. What would GP do?

I also take comfort from some of the world's great religions. Staying at a Zen Buddhist temple in Japan in 2016, I fasted with the resident monks for cycles of eighteen hours a day, having a six-hour eating window (no breakfast, lunch at 11.30am, dinner at 5.30pm). For some Catholics, such as my father as a child in the early '60s, fasting occurred prior to receiving Communion, starting at midnight on Saturday before Sunday mass. (At Catholic dances on Saturday night, a late supper would be served in a nod to the fasting that would soon follow.) The communal aspect of the fasts is appealing. I feel quite isolated on my detox. I want to go through this hardship with others.

There are lots of blogs on how to get through Ramadan without gnawing your arm off. I like the set-up: you are all in it together – being hungry, getting irritable, thinking about food between sunrise and sunset, but the greater glory is God. It means more than just detoxing your own body, which is necessarily a singular and solipsistic pursuit that seems more about disconnection and punishment than enlightenment. During Ramadan you break the fast together – in large, late-night suppers.

It is hard detoxing on your own, particularly in a city as obsessed with food as Sydney.

For the first few days I feel exhausted and am sleeping a lot. When I return from the fasting clinic and lie down for a minute or two, I wake hours later, foggy and confused – a jet-laggy, displaced feeling of not knowing if I've woken at the start of the day or the middle of night. I listen as the suburb goes about its business – the cries of the lorikeets from the fig trees, a backpacker sitting under a large tree outside my room strumming Jeff Buckley on a banjo, bottles of wine clinking in plastic bags and people laughing, on their way to a party.

When the hunger wakes me at 4am, growling, my stomach clenching, I prowl the flat. It's one of those solid, lovely 1950s blocks – faded Florence Broadhurst wallpaper in the lobby, thick walls and high ceilings, strangely shaped rooms, a hexagon-tiled bathroom and a sunroom that looks down over the roofs of Bondi to the beach. To fill myself up, I drink water, make cups of tea and squirt in a juicy portion of honey to cut through the bitterness.

Writing distracts from the hunger. Sometimes writing focuses me on the hunger. The moon floods over my writing desk and I sit and scribble notes. *My nose is running like I have a bad cold.* And: *Dreamt I was a horse midwife – again.*

I drift around the place. My jaw aches – a strange feeling, like a toothache. In my mouth there is a feeling of absence – like I'm missing all my teeth. But in reality, my teeth are missing food. Their only real job is to chew stuff and now they are useless, just sort of there, hanging out in my mouth. In the kitchen, when I'm sure my housemate, Jo, is asleep, I stand by the sink and masticate but don't swallow stuff that I can literally sink my teeth into – cardboard, plastic, bubble wrap – just so I can keep them in action, fit for duty for when I return to eating. I'm aware of how this looks and I don't want to be seen.

On day three there is a shift in gear for the worse. The low-level depression has mostly lifted and in its place is … nothing, a blank. I'm a zombie, someone with not enough energy to feel depressed. I stare out windows. I stare *at* windows. I cannot concentrate. I remember I have to do something but then forget a minute or so later what that something is. My brain is foggy – that superb, mysterious engine that I take for granted, that has got me all my jobs, that is responsible for keeping me in cash to buy interesting shoes and lattes and mid-priced champagne – is now spluttering to a standstill. I need to keep writing articles to pay my rent but I can't remember the password for my computer, let alone how to pick up the phone or structure a story. I don't get how people do this fast while working. It takes me fifteen minutes just to put on my socks.

Now I understand why some people on heavy sedatives plead to come off them, preferring ragged madness to the sort of stupefied, glassy world they inhabit on the pills. I spend hours in the too-warm house, the plastic fan blades turning, staring out the window at the thin blue line of the ocean in the distance. It's a Rothko painting or positive pregnancy test and I'm a lobotomised patient – like the young woman in Sylvia Plath's *The Bell Jar*, with her 'perpetual marble calm'. Thoughts are not quite forming, like water about to boil. There are almost bubbles, something is about to rise to the surface; it's trying to get there really, really hard … but not quite yet. My eyeballs have been replaced by stones, my tongue is furry and useless and heavy – imagine a carpet that's been left out in the rain.

My brain during this time is ravenous. Usually the brain uses 20 per cent of the body's resting energy expenditure (so, calories) – but takes glycogen (sugar) as fuel. It won't use amino acids, which are broken down from proteins, or fatty acids and glycerol, which are broken down from fats. As a back-up it can switch to ketone bodies, produced by the liver from fatty acids during periods of fasting, low- or no-carbohydrate diets, starvation and intense exercise. This metabolic switch to ketone bodies takes several days. After fasting for three days, the brain gets 30 per cent of its energy from ketone bodies. After four days, this goes up to 75 per cent.

This is where I am – stalled like a car on the side of the road, yet to switch gear to the ketones. Maybe because of this lack of fuel, I'm sleeping a lot. It seems the best way through this early 'shock' phase of the fast. Without caffeine artificially geeing me up and alcohol and other soporifics bringing me down, my body is finding its natural resting rhythm – which seems to be to sleep for sixteen to eighteen hours a day.

Blogs from other fasters talk about sleeping a lot. Everyone just takes to their cots in the hard early days of the fast. The bloggers reckon they are sleepy because the body is pulling energy from where it can in order to kick off its mammoth cleaning and detox effort.

I speak to Associate Professor Amanda Salis from the University of Sydney, who leads research and multidisciplinary clinical trials at the Boden Institute of Obesity, Nutrition, Exercise and Eating Disorders. Her research focuses on understanding and circumventing the body's responses to ongoing energy restriction, a phenomenon she terms the 'famine reaction'. She says the reason I am sleeping so much is that 'your body goes into conservation mode when you are fasting. There is not enough fuel to enable your muscles to move. Neurochemical changes are occurring in your brain, also making you feel lethargic. It's like being hit by a train.' Indeed.

Sleeping also makes time go by. It relieves the tedium. But even sleep does not bring relief. The texture of my sleep has become strange – viscous, its fathoms so deep I get the bends coming up in the morning. I've always been a dreamer, spending those first few moments of consciousness trying to hold on to the tail ends of dreams – the unlikely scenarios, the jumble of places, the emotional weather of each scene. But fasting is taking my dream life to a different, higher and scarier level. It's as if, bereft of stimulation, my subconscious is busy creating the most freaky, scary horror show each and every night.

Coursing through everything is anxiety. I am running from gate lounge to gate lounge trying to find the gate for my departure to Barkly. Where is Barkly? What is Barkly? I don't know but I have to go there. I run onto the tarmac but they won't let me get on the plane.

The dreams seem so real that my life undergoes a curious kind of inversion. Dreams are more vivid than my actual life, crowded with big emotion and drama, brilliant, teeming and terrifying, while my waking life is non-time in which my brain, slowing right down without any fuel, is having trouble making connections. I'm thinking of the name for that thing – you know the thing – the thing you boil water in – what's it called? It's in the kitchen next to the toaster.

And all the while there is still the hunger. The brilliant British essayist George Orwell writes in *Down and Out in Paris and London*, 'Hunger reduces one to an utterly spineless, brainless condition, more like the after-effects of influenza than anything else. It is as though one had been turned into a jellyfish, or as though all one's blood had been pumped out and lukewarm water substituted.' Orwell's 'hunger mentor', his friend Boris, provides this advice: 'It is fatal to look hungry. It makes people want to kick you.'

I am still under self-imposed house arrest. They can't kick you if they can't see you, and I have retreated deep into this corner of Bondi – the bed pushed up against the wall, its soft tangle of white sheets, its pink floral summer quilt – in the small room in the ground-floor flat, where no one can find me.

All the wellness blogs say days three and four are the worst. And so it comes to pass.

I have a sore lower back. My fevered, glucose-starved brain is craving answers – and the answers I find are on the internet. Steve Hendricks in *Harper's* says that lower back pain is common with fasters, and that many believe it's caused by toxins exiting the body, although there is little evidence to support this hypothesis.

So maybe it's all the unprocessed drugs now leaving my tissue – the decades-old ecstasy tablets, or Valiums, or the diet pills I misused to help me finish my novel, the Panadols, Naprogesics, the antimalarials or the blood pressure medication. In the sweat and stink of my mid-afternoon fugue (the twist of the dampening sheets, the fetid floral summer quilt) I imagine the inside of my body. It's 2007 in there, eternally 3am, and I'm still in the club in Shoreditch. The half a tab of ecstasy I took is finally ready, many years later, to make its journey out of my body. It's been trapped in a tissue – where? – somewhere in there, for all this time. But now its moment has arrived. The fast and its mysterious forces have pulled the chemical compound into my bloodstream, and it's recirculating through my body like a partly activated landmine or a roused sleeper cell. I am not getting high. I am not loving everyone and waving my arms in the air like I just don't care. This is the mother of all comedowns.

The back pain can also – says the internet – be a reactivation of an old injury or illness. Could it be a weird echo from the past? I'd been hospitalised for an untreated UTI that turned into a kidney infection fifteen years before, when I was living in Dublin. Now in Bondi, so many years later, I recognised the pain. Hello, old friend. It was dull and tender, like I'd been badly bruised on the inside, like a muscle strain in my lower back, but deeper.

Is this what the fasters on the internet call a 'healing crisis'? They say that fasting dissolves or expels diseased tissue in the body – say, from the site of an old injury – and redistributes nutrients. In other words, I'm being healed and cleaned from the inside. Which is a less metaphorical explanation of exactly what Jared Six described: during a long fast, the body is like a store closed for clean-up and stocktake.

But what if the joint and muscle pain is not a healing crisis but a sign of malnutrition? Health websites such as LiveStrong and MedlinePlus take this view: 'Muscle pains and aches may be caused by malnourishment and insufficient levels of nutrients. In particular, potassium and calcium deficiencies can cause muscle pains due to an imbalance of electrolytes.'

This malnutrition explanation for physical pain clashes with the almost romantic thesis on the fasting blogs – that past injuries and hurts are being healed.

Associate Professor Amanda Salis is also sceptical of the notion of a healing crisis. She puts it viscerally:

When you are fasting or eating very little, your body is
eating itself from the inside out. It eats up bones, muscles
and organs for energy. It takes a chomp out of your liver
and spleen, and in terms of whether fasting uses up dead
tissues – these tissues would be eliminated anyway. A
healing crisis sounds like something people would say to
make you feel better psychologically when your body is
fighting back against starvation – a condition your body
responds to in a life-or-death manner, because your body
knows that fasting or semi-fasting will eventually result
in death.

I am taking in around 250 calories a day with the herbs – so the
body does have some nutrients and energy coming in. But if you go
long enough without food, the ultimate risk is death by starvation.

When all you have left is your body – when it is your only form
of protest, the only instrument of your agency – you can starve it,
or cut it, or set it alight. Your body is yours and if in the detention
centre, the hospital or the prison, they take away the sheets and
the razor blades, the pills and the plastic bags, you can refuse to
eat if you want to slip out, if you want to do it on your own terms.
Fasting kills.

In the 1950s and '60s, fasting was used as an experimental
treatment for obesity, and several patients died from heart failure.

In 2010, a woman in Florida died from heart failure after
twenty-one days of fasting. According to a report in 2017 in the
British Medical Journal, a 47-year-old woman was admitted to hospital, suffering from seizures brought on by low sodium levels
in her blood. She had been on a 'herbal medication' detox, also

drinking vast amounts of water, green tea and sage. She recovered once her sodium levels returned to normal.

In 1981 Irish political prisoners went on a hunger strike, protesting the British presence in Northern Ireland. Ten prisoners – including their leader, Bobby Sands – died after periods of between forty-six and seventy-three days without food.

At the age of seventy-four and already skinny, Mahatma Gandhi survived twenty-one days of total starvation, only allowing himself sips of water.

Doctors treating patients with anorexia nervosa found death from organ failure or heart attack is fairly common (up to 20 per cent of cases end this way) and tends to happen when body weight has fallen to between 30 and 40 kilograms, corresponding to a body mass index (BMI) approximately half of normal. Unless other causes intervene, a patient with end-stage cancer often dies after losing 35–45 per cent of their body weight.

But the science is inexact. According to the *Scientific American*, mortality rates vary enormously depending on size, metabolism and other factors, such as any pre-existing illness.

Even if you don't die, the website Quackwatch says, 'People who survive prolonged fasts (starvation) may suffer anemia, decreased immunity, osteoporosis, kidney damage, or liver damage. Depressed gastrointestinal or digestive functions may persist for weeks or months. The worst thing about fasting is its destruction of lean and vital tissue needed for a healthy and active life.'

My body thinks this *will eventually result in death*. It doesn't know when this starvation will end. It doesn't differentiate between doing this for a magazine assignment and a Northern

Irish hunger strike. So was I being healed? Or was I making myself very ill and dicing with death?

Albert Einsten once said, 'An empty stomach is not a good political adviser.' Maybe it is my fuzzy brain, but things other than logic are taking over my decision-making. Vanity, I'm sure. I am dropping dress sizes at an alarming clip. But faith also wins out over logic. I somehow believe the blogs and testimonials. I cling to the idea of a healing crisis. It allows me to remove myself from the horror and mystery of what is going on in my body, and instead take on the role of harsh but fair nurse. 'Yes,' I say to my body, 'this is painful, but it's for your own good.'

After spending all day lying in my disgusting bed, I smell something incredible. My housemate, Jo, has cooked bacon in a large pan. The pan is on the stove. Jo cooks wonderful food and had kindly offered to move out of the house for the duration of the fast, so that the apartment would be a totally food-free and therefore temptation-free zone. But Jo had already had to move out once, temporarily, when I contracted whooping cough and, as a public-health risk, was quarantined at home. Being a stoic I assured her that I would not be tempted, not one little bit, even if she cooked multi-course dinner parties consisting mostly of bacon. And no – the smell of the coffee brewing in the morning, that is really nothing that would tempt me. No siree, not at all. Baking a cake? Go for it! So Jo stayed and cooked and I crept into the kitchen when she was gone and pressed my nose to a fresh baguette as furtively as a pervert.

But right now I am in agony because she's cooked bacon in the pan. She's cooked bacon in the pan. How on earth could she be so cruel as to cook bacon in the pan? I put my head close to it and breathe in a whisper of the scent, a fading bacon vapour trail. That it's congealed and yellowed fails to deter me. It's such an attractive foodstuff. Bacon is *so incredible*. I wonder if she truly appreciated the bacon. If she truly appreciated how fucking great bacon is.

I look around cautiously and run my tongue along the base of the pan. I feel every bump of every crusted-on bit of whatever it is that is stuck there. It's like I am tongue-kissing a gross giant with a rough mouth: tongue to tongue, gritty, thick, salty, oily, knobbly and gobby. Oh man, I just long to feel something. It's been ninety hours without food.

After that shameful moment, I devise a work-around. I tell myself I can put stuff in my mouth; the key is not to swallow. As the week goes on, my behaviour starts to resemble that of a person with an eating disorder. I am obsessed with food, but petrified of swallowing lest it ruin the mysterious alchemy of the fast. (Dr Liu said I can't even chew gum.)

I grab chunks of meat Jo has cooked, chew then spit them in the bin. I lick a gravy pan because I crave flavour. I email Mum to let her know how I am faring. She replies, *Please DO NOT lick the juices from pans. You could burn your tongue.* With my enhanced sense of smell, I am drawn into a Japanese restaurant. I cave and buy some wonderful-smelling gyozas. I do not intend to eat the gyozas, just chew on them. I ram them into my mouth, masticate and spit the undigested lump into a bin. I hope I have not been seen by anyone I know.

Each night I call my parents and ask them to describe what they are cooking for dinner, what they had for lunch and any snacks they might have enjoyed that day. I particularly like hearing about their cocktail hour – aperitivo at 6pm, neighbours over for a drink or two and some cheese, the table set outside, the mist from the Southern Ocean rolling in from the dunes. It seems healthy, civilised, a proper way to live – rather than drinking a mystery sludge three times a day, sleeping for eighteen hours and spitting food into bins.

At first my parents are flattered by my interest in the minutiae of their meals. I've never listened so keenly to them before, never showed such interest in their nutrition or dietary habits. Such keen, keen interest! As a child, I hid portions of vegetables in my sleeve or spat them out into napkins. But now I long for those childhood stems of steamed broccoli, the mashed pumpkin and potato. On the phone, Mum reels off every ingredient in the salad she has just prepared, Dad describes the different meats he is barbecuing. I ring them after dinner too, just to see how their meal worked out – did they enjoy it? What did their guests think? What did their guests bring? What did they prefer – the lamb chop or the rump steak? Then one night they suddenly stop elaborating, sensing something off. They are terse: 'Yes, dinner was fine, thanks for asking. We had a barbecue.' There is something wrong with these long, lovely conversations about food, something unwholesome. I am like the panting man on a phone-sex call, begging for a detailed description of acts from which I was excluded and – far away, in a lonely bedroom – getting off on it.

In addition to deep fatigue, listlessness, headaches, hunger and obsessiveness about food, in the first week of the fast I have what feels like a big dip in blood pressure. I guess it's better than having dangerously high blood pressure. When I stand up from bed or a chair, I get dizzy and have to clutch at something, so as not to fall.

This occurs because fasting causes blood sugar levels to drop. My body has lost water, sodium and potassium, which produces a condition called postural hypotension (low blood pressure when standing up). Forget dying from starvation or heart attack. Right now, my greatest risk is cracking my skull after fainting.

When walking around the flat, I stay close to the walls, my palm pressed flat to them in case of sudden vertigo. I cling on to the handrail in the shower, like an old person – frail and liable to fall.

On day four of the detox, I am almost killed. It's the hump day of the fast, according to all the literature. In his pamphlet Dr Liu writes in his usual understated way: 'In general patients find days 4 to 7 of the first 14 days of treatment are the most difficult days.' My friend Patrick is picking me up to go for a swim and I am almost hit by a car and then another car as I try to cross the road to meet him. Patrick is waving his arms at me, begging me not to cross the road and yelling frantically that he'll bring the car around. *He never brings the car around*, I think several seconds later, after I almost get run over for a third time as I turn to cross back and narrowly avoid being struck by the 380 bus. I am a beat behind myself. I am two beats behind the traffic.

Patrick urges me not to try to cross the road by myself until I break the fast and, apart from going to the fasting clinic every day, avoid leaving the house because of the way I smell and my general 'very weird, slightly scary demeanour'.

When we get to the beach, I swim and clutch my jaw, the ache more pronounced in the salt water. It's like someone has punched me, or I have a gum infection or a mouthful of rotting teeth (perhaps it is the pain of my teeth, missing food, reminding me that they are still there).

So that's it for a while. I just go between home and the clinic. The clinic and home. And after a while, the people at the clinic – Dr Liu's Chinese workers – become my only friends. And I love them all, really I do. The clinic is only closed one day a year, on Christmas Day, and many of the workers appear to be there seven days a week. My favourite is an older, stooped woman. She doesn't speak English, so we mainly rely on exaggerated facial expressions to communicate. Talking to her is like texting someone using emoji. Sometimes she claps and looks unfathomably delighted when I lose weight. She'll slap me on the arse and giggle, and record my kilograms in a ledger. But she's not always high octane. Sometimes she gives me lacklustre stomach massages, and when I sneak open my eyes, her gaze is elsewhere, staring at the wall. She's lifting up and putting down bits of my midriff flesh like it's dough, and she's making her twentieth loaf of sourdough for the day.

Then there is Peter (which I am sure is not his actual Chinese name), who has the best English of all the workers. He is getting his Chinese medicine qualifications at the University of Technology Sydney. Most of the Chinese doctors in China are studying Western medicine, he says. 'Only a few people do Chinese medicine, but they are out in the countryside.' They are the pre-moderns, the ancients left over from the Time of the Needles. It's only the very wealthy Australians, in this wedge of Sydney, who are creating the demand for Chinese doctors, the healers with maps of meridian lines on their office doors, the chakra realigners, the energy cleansers, the apothecaries with their mystery medicine made of roots and leaves.

Peter leaves for a while to visit his mum back in China. When he comes back, he reels off the incredible delights she fed him – the wontons (oh, wanton wontons!), dumplings, fried rice, roast duck – oblivious to the fact that I am literally starving. (Tell me more, I beg him – were the dumplings pork and were they steamed or fried? And when you had the stopover in Singapore did you have chilli mud crab at that place at Changi Airport, you know the one?)

There is also a group of older, severe, non-English-speaking male clinicians. I get to know them by their touch. Each has a different hand pressure, and each is brilliant and precise. But I can never relax into the massages – they are too gruelling. The bruises that dot my body are in the shape of their fingerprints.

After the massage they put a dozen needles in my forehead and scalp and across my stomach, which becomes black and blue with bruises big and small. 'Sorry, stomach; sorry, old bean,' I whisper when they leave the room. 'You've served me well. You've made room, uncomplainingly, for all those pies. And this is how I reward you.' Peter tells me the acupuncture is to get rid of the headaches I am experiencing and to calm me down so I can sleep (but sleep is all I do!). The needles on the stomach are to assist my organs achieve optimum function. I'm not sure why they put needles in my legs. Maybe something to do with meridian lines. According to some fasting blogs, that is where a lot of pain of the detox is felt – in the legs. Towards the end of a week of this, there is no part of my stomach that doesn't look like a bouquet of cabbage flowers: purples and pinks, bright, florid and tender with bruises.

By day five without food, there is no hiding from the truth: I smell bad. Really bad. Not sweaty, but like something that's been left in the bin too long and is rotting.

At first, lying in bed on a beautiful sunny day, with the windows open and the breeze blowing in, I think a backpacker must have left chicken carcasses in the bins in the neighbouring park. *Revolting*, I think, *whoever left meat out to rot is gross*. (Or in my slow state of cognition, what I actually think is: *Smell meat bad, chicken, gross, rotting backpacker*.)

The smell is not dissimilar to an incident from my university days. I minded a friend's car when she went to Japan for the summer, but she took the keys with her, unfortunately locking in a tray of meat I had accidentally left under the seat. It cooked in the car all summer, through a string of those dry, shimmering Melbourne days when the temperature doesn't dip below 40 degrees. The smell was first unignorable, then unimaginable. The whole street – a genteel Parkville cul-de-sac of rose gardens and renovated terraces, professors and paediatric surgeons – seemed to be clouded in the odour coming from our garage. The meat rotted through the rubber mat and then the metal floor of the car. The RACV people had to come over in hazard suits to unlock the vehicle.

That is what I am smelling now. Rotting meat. It's grim. After closing my bedroom window I realise with horror that the rotting smell has not gone away. It is worse. And it is coming from within me. Even my tears smell bad.

Is this part of the cleaning process, I wonder? I ask Associate Professor Amanda Salis about this odour. She says, 'Bad breath is associated with fasting. This is partly due to ketones. There is also less hydration of the mouth, so saliva is not replenished. Skin cells in your mouth rot by bacteria that produce gases that smell bad.'

She can't explain my whole-body smell.

Dr Liu warned of smells in his materials, which I am now consulting constantly: 'You may have bad breath because your body is releasing toxins, you could brush your teeth as many times as you like, but no chewing gum.' The pamphlet is silent on the issue of body odour. I apply expensive lotions to my skin and start showering more than once a day, but nothing is removing the smell.

This fast has turned me into a bedroom depressive with very little in the way of social engagements (no one wants to hang out with you when you are not eating) but I resolve to have no contact with anybody while I smell like this. People will gag – possibly vomit – if I get too close. I decide that when I am forced to interact with someone, I will stand at least 50 metres away from them and shout, or communicate via text message. The fasting clinic staff don't count because the clinic itself has a weird smell.

Despite smelling like an open drain, being foggy in the head, feeling constantly miserable and listless, behaving in a disgusting and weird way in public, having bloodshot eyes and doing strange things late at night (I have been chewing pantry items and then spitting the ball of stuff into the bin and putting heaps of tissues over the clump of masticated food – a trick used by anorexics) and almost being killed by traffic – I am getting thinner! Much thinner!

By day six I have lost 5.3 kilograms. It's the most weight I have ever lost in one go. The weight is coming off my face, my chest, my stomach and my thighs. I am shrinking, like a grape turning into a sultana.

While I should feel pleased that the fast is having one of its desired effects, my life is the most boring it's ever been. I can't focus on anything on TV for longer than ten minutes and I can't concentrate on reading unless it's cookbooks, which I stare at – not reading so much as horsily inhaling pictures of super-stylised food in a sort of magical thinking that equates gazing to grazing. The body will find a way through one of its senses. If it can't taste it will smell and if it can't smell it will gaze – like the thirsty stare reserved for someone you desire but can never have. I have recently read David Foster Wallace's *The Pale King*. He was doing the hard sell on boredom in that novel, convinced it was the road to bliss. It was just like the icy mountain pass – you only reached nirvana once you moved through it. He wrote that 'dullness is associated with psychic pain' because it doesn't provide enough stimulation to distract people from the deeper pain 'that's always there'.

So here I am, just me and the dullness and its evil cousin, psychic pain. In those weeks when I am fasting, the spectre of meaninglessness lurks everywhere. I wonder if it has been there all along, covered up with food 'n' stuff – or if it is making its first appearance. You see, once you take everything away – the shopping and the eating, the preparing and the cleaning up, the cooking and the cafes, the friends and the restaurants and the parties and the drinks (all the drinks!), the quiet morning coffee with the paper in the sun, the barista who knows your name and the barman who reads your mood, the celebrations and the dates, the routines and the rituals – once you throw all that away, a sort of hush descends. In it you can see and feel and know the emptiness that is in the room before the room where the meaninglessness resides. In its bland way, it's quite terrifying.

start to have serious doubts about the fast towards the end of the first week, when I am woken at 1am by a sensation that feels like a heart attack. There are sharp, shooting pains in my chest on the left side that eventually settle to small but very alarming electrical pulsations. Is it bad enough to go to the hospital? I google 'heart attack'. Yes, I can move my arm and count backwards from ten, but this feeling moving across my torso is unlike anything I have ever experienced. It's very unpleasant, like something electronic has been implanted in my chest and is malfunctioning.

Despite my concern, there is an overriding emotion: embarrassment. I picture rocking up to Emergency and telling them that I haven't eaten for six days. No, it's not a political act. And I'm not mentally ill. I don't have an eating disorder. It's for a magazine assignment – I'm a gonzo wellness journalist! I start to wonder if what I am doing is a form of self-harm. To reduce my anxiety I practise deep breathing and sit up until dawn, too scared to go to sleep in case I don't wake up. In the morning I text Dr Liu. He replies straightaway that there's no need to worry, that I should just come in for my usual one-hour treatment – which I do, ragged, anxious and wild-eyed, not sure whether to trust my instincts or him.

Despite my scare with chest pains, I push on. I feel like I've come this far, and I may as well keep going. It's New Year's Eve and I am lying in a hot tub in a backyard in Newtown. The baby, Otis, is sleeping upstairs, his parents at a party on the harbour. In the backstreets all around me are the sounds of people ringing in the new year. There is a bloom of fireworks, then the sky is still, poised, like any moment it might tear open in a storm. I can smell the eucalyptus from the old gum trees in the heady, heavy, rain-scented air. Around midnight, I open the fridge and see the week-old, still-juicy Christmas ham wrapped in cloth and the mince pies and chocolates. *Happy New Year.* I close the fridge. I open the fridge. I close the fridge.

Later, I'm pulled back there by hunger and boredom. *I'll just take a look*, I tell myself. The light is on, and my hand and arm up to the elbow is in the fridge, deep in the middle cavity, like a surgeon operating inside a crowded abdomen. I see a tub of hummus, open the lid and run my index finger through it. It's been six days without food. On my tongue the hummus is like none I've ever tasted. This simple, supermarket hummus is creamy and nutty, fluffy and unctuous. My mouth floods with saliva. As Seneca wrote to Lucilius in 65AD, 'You will leap for joy when filled with a pennyworth of food.'

I keep my finger in my mouth a long time after the hummus has melted on my tongue, until all that's left is the memory of the memory of the taste.

So it's come to this.

**

Around me, life happens. I have a book coming out. It's my first novel. It only took eight years to write. My publisher rings me, very excited: the director of the Sydney Writers' Festival, Jemma Birrell, is interested in putting my novel in the festival program. She wants to meet me first – just to see, I suppose, that I am normal, that she can put me on a panel without incident. I don't tell my publisher that I haven't eaten for a week now, and haven't been near a cafe for fear of breaking the fast.

'Refeeding syndrome' is an anxiety in the fasting community and can prove more dangerous than the fast itself. Be cavalier with your first meal, and it could be your last.

An *Associated Press* report from 28 August 1929 told of the death of forty-year-old Chris Solbert following a month-long fast, which he broke by consuming several beef sandwiches. I find other anecdotes on the wellness sites – people who broke their fasts with chocolate biscuits and got incredibly ill, a guy who ate a meal of beefsteak, potatoes, bread and butter and coffee after twenty-seven days of fasting. He was seized with violent vomiting spells.

The body goes through biological changes when it is fasting, including a slowing-down of the production of enzymes used to break down food. Introducing food slowly allows the body time to re-establish this enzyme production, as well as build up the lining of mucus in the gut.

With this in mind – and aware that I am about to enter a cafe that will be cooking bacon – I get a taxi to Jeds in North Bondi. Jemma orders breakfast and three lattes (not at once, she staggers her order). I'm trying to be normal, talking about my book. I cannot make eye contact with her while she is eating; it's sure to send me over the edge. I'm telling her about my novel – a group of murderous teens at an elite university college – 'wotevs, blah, blah, blah, some shit like that,' I'm saying, but I'm looking over at the door. I can smell her food. I can smell her coffee. I wonder if she can smell me detoxing. Hopefully she has a cold or blocked nose. I wonder how everyone in this cafe can eat so much food. People who are largely sedentary are tucking into enormous plates of bacon and eggs, toast and avocado. It's like they're nineteenth-century farm workers who have to use scythes and ploughs over large tracts of land. But what are these people really *doing*? Maybe a yoga class, maybe a short stroll around the farmers' market, but not actual *farming*.

Jemma turns to order her third coffee. As she does, a reptilian aspect of my brain takes over. This is pure biology, basic and urgent – the need to hunt, kill and eat. I simply must eat. Jemma's saying, 'Latte, extra hot, soy, in a takeaway cup,' and I'm reaching over, my hand taking on the shape of an eagle's claw. My fist lands on her plate and I scoop up a handful of tomato, some eggs, a crust, and jam it into my mouth. She turns back and sees it all in a horrified instant – her half-eaten food in my hand, almost missing my mouth in the haste, bits smeared on my chin, some of it dropping into my collar and the moan of pleasure, when at last, after a week, I swallow.

I've always been a social animal. I'm an extrovert who gets my energy from being around people. I love going out, I love gatherings and conversation and parties – just being with other people. During my fast it is apparent how much socialising (probably 90 per cent, in my case) takes place over food and drink. The isolation of the fast is hard going. In *Down and Out in Paris and London*, Orwell said the worst aspect of hunger was boredom. That and the sense that when you take food away, you take some essential human dignity away. 'You discover that a man who has gone even a week on bread and margarine is not a man any longer, only a belly with a few accessory organs.'

By the end of week one, I'm going out of my mind. It has been boring, but also incredibly self-absorbed. The clinic staff and I attend to my body as if it is some fragile holy relic to be studied and turned over, applying mysterious treatments to restore it to some glorious past. (Did my body ever have a glorious past? Maybe when I was a child?) To quote writer David Rakoff, who fasted to find enlightenment: 'My days are taken up in this narcissistic rumination about intake and output ... This is one of the most self-obsessed things I have ever done in my life. And I say this as a first-person journalist.'

When I feel strong enough to go out and not eat (not steal food, or lick food, or spit chewed-up food into public bins), I make arrangements to meet a friend for dinner. Chris is coming to Sydney and wants to go out in Kings Cross. It would be ridiculous not to see him. Chris used to meet me for lunch in Melbourne; lunches that would roll into cocktails then supper, glasses of wine into bottles, bottles into more bottles. We hopped from rooftop bar to rooftop bar, the ones where you could smoke. There were nights when the city blazed and things sped up like in a time-lapse video: there's the Princess Bridge at dusk, the Yarra at night, all inky and black, the small bar above Degraves Street and the restaurant with the door under the stairs, credit cards thrown down, change not collected. We talk and talk and talk and talk, and never have to go home if we don't want to.

How different this night is. He orders beer and I order water. He orders dinner and I order nothing. It's weird. The vibe is off.

I have underestimated how uncomfortable people feel when they are eating and drinking and you are not. If you don't eat together it unbalances the dynamic profoundly. I wonder if there is something deep in our DNA that makes us distrust someone who will not break bread with us. Perhaps there's an ancient, primal fear of being poisoned that means we only relax if everyone is eating the same food – lest there be an assassin in our midst.

The fast has also been the longest I have ever gone without alcohol since I was a teenager – and one of the things I will have to learn as I emerge from my stinky-bedroom day-sleeper solitude is how to socialise without booze.

But my night with Chris turns out all right. We talk. He eats and has a couple of beers. I cave and have a small teaspoon of rice. Our friendship doesn't fall apart because we aren't drinking together. It turns out something great built on nights of a thousand cocktails is still pretty great if you take away the cocktails. Which gets me thinking: is relying on alcohol for connections and closeness a bit like using a crutch when there's nothing wrong with your legs?

My whole way of living has been thrown into stark relief by the drama and extremity of the fast. The revelations are a mixture of the banal and profound: life is short, but even shorter if you don't look after your health. I notice that when something upsets me I have an immediate craving for something hot and salty – like a dim sim! – and that I and most people I know eat double the amount of calories we actually need. And that 70 per cent of what we eat is just habit. And that the reason people on a diet are mean and short-tempered is that it's miserable being hungry all the time. And this:

the hedonism jag I've been on is fun but exhausting, and maybe it's time to pull up stumps. My health, with high blood pressure and cholesterol, is not going to be robust forever. But how to regulate? My modus operandi before the fast was to go out a lot – five or six nights a week – then enjoy a day or two of solitude to balance the socialising. Now it's all solitude. I am beginning to hate it. Some balance is needed. I'm tired of being on such an extreme treadmill.

In the long, long empty hours of the fast, I pass the time by fantasising about how I'm going to live when I can go back on solids. I imagine myself as someone others might find inspiring: serene, clean, lean, able to make one glass of wine (good wine, expensive wine) last all night. I'm the sort of person who has small portions of good food, who doesn't emotionally eat or buy dim sims when she is stressed. 'How do you do it?' my dining companions would ask, awed. 'Well,' I would answer, waving away the bread basket, 'many years ago, I did an extreme fast, I didn't eat for weeks. But I learnt a lot – about myself, my body and society.' I would smile with gleaming teeth, my hands folded over my flat stomach, and take a teeny-tiny sip of wine.

It isn't that I want to be thin. If I turn this fantasy over in my hands, what I really want is self-control, and to be admired for that self-control. What I am now is the opposite – I have no control, I'm a can't-say-no hedonist. And I don't know whether I am admired for that, or pitied. But I know I think about myself in contradictory terms: *this is fun, keep partying* – and – *oh God, this shit is getting old. When are you going to stop?*

B
y day eight I have lost six kilograms and loads of inches. Gone are five inches from my stomach and one to three inches from my arms, thighs, waist and hips. Dr Liu is happy with my progress. He says I'm on track, and if I keep going with the program, following it to the letter, my organs will be able to breathe again and return to their optimum function. I will achieve my goal of being clean.

As well as losing weight, I'm starting to look different. Gone is the swollen and bloated look of my face, the boozy pallor, the cloudy eyes. I am beginning to look – there is no other term for it – obscenely healthy. That summer, sorting out boxes in my parents' garage, I find photos of me in my twenties. Fifteen years later I look better. I look *younger*.

My hair is super shiny and my nails are strong. They used to peel, break off and bend but now they seem built from different, tougher material. I could open tins with these bad boys. But the weirdest is my skin. I didn't have a lot of wrinkles (I was starting to believe that all the alcohol and processed foods had had a sort of pickling effect on my face – preserving it in a creepily youthful way) but there were definitely some. But now my face – my thinner face – is taut, shiny and very, very smooth. The lines around my eyes, my mouth and my forehead have just disappeared, pretty much overnight. This freaks me out a lot. Where have they gone? How can wrinkles just disappear? Don't laboratories around the world spend billions of dollars trying to do this? I had thought wrinkles were irreversible without surgery. Is it all the sleep I'm getting? My eyes are strangely bright, and my sense of smell has sharpened. Down on level one of Bondi Junction, I can smell the dead-animal woodland odour of Dr Liu's on level four.

With this new face and body, I rejoin the Sydney hoi polloi. I meet Patrick at the opening night of the Sydney Festival. He hasn't seen me since I was blotchy-faced and red-eyed, a high risk of pedestrian death on Bondi Road. There is free booze but I'm not tempted. When you give up food, trust me – booze is the last thing you crave. I want chips, pizza, oranges, spinach, steak, potato gratin, tortilla chips, mashed potato – not fizzy wine in a plastic cup.

I am looking thin(ish) for the first time since I was a child. I am wearing a pretty red low-cut dress that nips in at my new, shrinking waist and my hair is blow-dried. I have a flower tucked behind my ear. Patrick looks me up and down. 'You look … hmmmm. Like, what is it? A skinny eastern-suburbs PR chick. Just like everyone else.'

I feel deflated in more ways than one. In getting thinner am I just going to look like everyone else in this part of Sydney?

Patrick sits down with a litre of beer and a foot-long German sausage with hot chips. When he goes to get mustard I grab a handful of his chips, put them in my mouth, lick them and put them back on his plate. They taste amazing but I haven't swallowed them – so I am still, officially, fasting. I tell Patrick not to eat the soggy chips on the side of his plate as they have been in my mouth. He shrugs, as if to say, 'girls and their diets', and pushes them off to one side.

How do other men react to the newer, thinner me? Thin is attractive, right? Yes? I look better – maybe the best I've ever looked. But it doesn't net me any additional male admirers. And the men I know already don't say much beyond a vague acknowledgement that I look 'different' or offering the non-compliment for elderly people: I look 'well'.

Instead it is mainly my female friends who are admiring of my weight loss. In me they see that if you bite down on your cheeks hard enough to stop the hunger, if you white-knuckle it, if you take your Chinese medicine thrice daily, if you lock up your pantry and don't leave your room, transformation is possible. Not just any old transformation, but radical, rapid transformation.

When I meet my friend Ellen in Hyde Park, she does a double take. She has been living in New York and the last time she saw me, I was lining up for a Shake Shack bacon burger in Madison Square Gardens. She can't stop staring. 'OMG, you look amazing – right now, just now – amazing. Your hair, your eyes, your skin! You need to stay looking like this. Just keep doing whatever it is you're doing.'

'But I'm really hungry. I miss going out for dinner. I miss socialising. I miss eating. I'm going to go back on solids soon, I can't wait to eat ...' I reel off all the foods I can't *wait* to eat including pasta, burgers, pho, salads, apples, granola, falafel, roast chicken. But she is shaking her head. 'No, Brig, you don't understand – you can't go back to eating, you are at peak hotness *now*.'

My friend Zoe, an actress, tells me that when losing weight for a role, 'my female friends thought I looked amazing and I got so many compliments from women, but my husband thought I was looking too much like a child. He was very relieved when I put the weight back on and my boobs came back.'

In *Lolita*, Humbert Humbert says peak hotness for females is between ages nine and fourteen. For me, the peak is a smaller, more specific window – in the months from December to March when I am fasting. But it is unsustainable to keep this almost sprite-like glow, like one of the girls from Hanging Rock come back years later, having made some sort of connection with the spirit world – the whites of my eyes luminous like polished opals, skin glowing, complexion smooth like a child's. This is Nature at her most spooky and supernatural. Is this what happens when you get clean? No one seems to understand how it works at all.

The kilograms keep falling off: 850 grams one day, 1.2 kilograms the next, one kilogram the next. It's so rapid and strange that I feel disassociated from it. In the pantry I pick up a one-kilogram packet of rice. It's really heavy. I can barely believe that I am losing the equivalent of one of these from my body every day. Where does it go?

In the first week I had lost weight equivalent to an airline's carry-on baggage allowance, one of those bags on wheels that has some clothes, a couple of books, some toiletries – enough for a weekend away. I was *carrying carry-on*, distributed around my body – my arms, my stomach, my thighs, my arse, my face. No wonder moving is now easier.

This is the first time I actually turn my mind to the sheer effort my body was going through just to carry those extra kilograms.

Now I feel – well, lighter. Being more streamlined, I glide along rather than heave myself from place to place. I'd become used to heaving – I didn't even think about it. I have less stiffness in my joints. Activities such as yoga are much easier. I can twist into certain positions with greater ease than before, and I'm more agile, particularly when transitioning from one pose to another.

But it feels so weird to rapidly change body shape, like I've woken up in the wrong body. On a deep level, you get used to carrying yourself around as you are. You become accustomed to your dimensions. Your body learns the chair it will fit best in, the clothes that won't cling and the cut of a jacket that flatters, and that if you run too fast your tits will swing wildly around like soap in a sock. Until one day they don't – because there are less of them to swing.

My mind hasn't caught up to my new body so I'm not revelling in it; I'm more puzzled by it. It's as if I've taken off my massive, heavy Burberry trench coat (*ahh, that's better, shaking my shoulders free*). But is this new shape mine forever, or just something I've borrowed?

Other things are also shifting. I am a long-time sufferer of PMS – aches and pains, a day in bed curled around a hot water bottle. But when my period comes, these symptoms fail to appear. Amanda Salis says, 'With an extreme lack of food there's a dampening of active sex hormone levels and fertility is reduced. Historically, famines were very good at controlling population growth.'

So my period pain has eased up, but my reproductive capacity has fallen.

Week two rolls on. I had thought by now the fast would get easier, but day nine is horrible. My personal vibe is plummeting. I am moving around in a cloud of neg; I hate everyone and everything. I'm trying to write a profile of Hollywood star Margot Robbie. I met her for a pot of tea and toast at a hotel in the Flatiron District in Manhattan a few weeks ago, which now feels like a different lifetime. I look at the picture I took of her on my phone (her PR pouncing on me as I did, assuming the unauthorised shot would pop up on some website or magazine): no make-up, dewy skin, clear eyes and shiny blonde hair. I'd heard of Hollywood people existing in a permanent state of semi-fasting – how else could someone appear so eternally lovely? I feel a wave of animus and envy. I'm emanating what's commonly known as 'bad vibes'.

The fasting blogs call this a mental detox. Just as your body is purging, moving through its layers of toxins, so is the mind becoming clean. I cannot find any science to back this up, other than putting myself through it.

According to the personal account of fasting by blogger Falon Blanco, 'With extended fasts it is normal to also have strong emotional reactions that have been suppressed, as the body brings these to the surface also for healing . . . This can be a difficult period.'

Yes, it can be.

The mental detox is releasing stuff in the form of highly vivid nightmares. The nightmares are so real that when I am awake, I can't shake them off. *It really is* like everyone in my family died, just like they did in my dream on the eighth night of the fast when their car exploded in a fireball, incinerating everything in and around it including them (and I ran and I ran and I ran towards them, trying to warn them, but the heat was radiant and alive and could not be breached).

The wellness blogs tell me that at this point the detox is getting deeper, burning layers (burning years and years and years and years) away. I'm cleaning myself out. For decades I've poured alcohol, chemicals and all manner of processed food down my throat; the cleanse – this deeper bit – was always going to be an extremely rough ride. This is the bit of the renovation that gets really serious. The builders have brought the jackhammers in, they are ripping up the foundation, they are fixing all the plumbing, they've lifted off the roof. I am both the building and the tenant – I am being destroyed and rebuilt *and* trying to live in the house that is being torn down around me. All I can do is hold on tight as all the work continues at speed.

As well as running on very low energy, I have developed another gross side effect (turn away now if you are delicate): horrendous diarrhoea. *Where is this coming from?* I wonder, since I haven't had any food for ten days. Is this the food I've been storing in my gut for twenty years? Are these the burgers and fries of my misspent youth? I'm scared about what is coming out of me. It resembles river silt. I google 'fasting excrement' gingerly, then shut my browser, grossed out. There are pages and pages of poo selfies, an endless gallery of filth.

So many questions, so few answers. It's difficult not to be sceptical, not to be anxious. The fasting blogs with their talk of a healing crisis say the problem is actually the solution. My body is cleaning itself out from the inside. It's dumping loads of rubbish and toxins into my bloodstream, and until I can expel them, they are making me sick. Oh, how I ache! I should be celebrating how sick I am feeling – it's the detox working. But … really? Is it? Is it really? What if it's my body getting really sick because I've stopped feeding it? Maybe the sickness is my body being poisoned by the mysterious herbs. Dr Liu is my poisoner, the nameless workers his court. The organ pain I'm experiencing is occurring because there is something terribly wrong going on in my body. The rivers of silt coming out of me are also not a good, normal look. And what about those mysterious chest pains on the fifth night? I shiver at the memory of them, and those sweat-drenched, breath-holding hours until dawn. Every day I don't eat is a day where I am hurting myself. Don't all the wellness people say 'listen to your body'? My body is emitting a fortnight-long primal scream.

I swim at Bondi, my jaw aching – triggered again by the salt water, it seems. Nausea comes in waves. Waves come in waves. This is like the world's worst, most lingering hangover. I go to the fasting clinic at 5pm. Stretched out on the table I'm a mess, covered in sand and bruises, parts of me too sore to touch. My stomach is now one mass of bruises. My hips are black and blue. It looks ugly, like I have been punched repeatedly but on different days. Some bruises are vivid, strong and new; others are fading – they're more the colour of potatoes, a floury browny-white. Today I do not, cannot, make small talk with the staff. The man treating me is kind. He's one of the old-timers, and now he is being particularly careful with me, resting his hand very lightly on my knee in between placing the needles on my stomach and hips (where to place the needles? There is no square of skin not already livid and hurt). The staff must be able to read it – in our faces, on our bodies – when things get really bad. All I crave right now, apart from food, is a little bit of tenderness.

At the clinic, as usual, I get weighed. I've put on 100 grams overnight. Was it the two grains of rice I had? The two grains wouldn't have added up to 100 grams. Maybe a single gram – not 100. The next day, day ten, I put on another 100 grams. This frightens me. I am not eating – how can I be gaining weight?

I get home from the weigh-in and go straight to bed, where I fall into a really deep sleep. It's 6.30pm. Whatever is going on inside me is so intense that everything needs to shut down for the work to be done.

On day eleven I wake up, expecting the usual inertia – the bored, crusty feeling of spending too long in bed, being too weak to do anything else. But my concentration and energy levels are through the roof! I don't think I've ever felt so sharp. My brain is a Rolls Royce, purring and preening, just out of the factory, in mint condition.

The hunger has gone and the mental fog has cleared as if a stiff breeze has come along. Think of a massive mountain range entirely obscured by mist, and then the weather lifts. The mountain is revealed in all its crisp, complex detail.

Most of my new-found energy is of the mental kind. When I attempt to walk fifteen minutes down a hill from Bondi Junction to Bondi, I have to keep stopping to rest on park benches, like an old woman pushing one of those wheelie carts. But, oh, my brain! My brain can do anything – and at such speed, like superfast internet broadband. Just as you realise how unfit you used to be when you start exercising, I am having the same revelation with my brain. I don't believe the guff that we only use 10 per cent but now it's like my mind has been thoroughly rinsed, tuned and given extra component parts. Feeling this sharp is wonderful. Hangovers, fatigue, the foggy feeling you get after a big meal don't just affect your body, I'm coming to realise, they also affect your mind and how it functions. I'm pretty certain that a lot of this weight I'm losing will come back after my fast but I want to keep this brain – this lovely, clean, clear, superfast brain.

This is the result of ketones in action. My body has switched over to a different fuel system – potentially a more efficient fuel system than the carbohydrates it was relying on for all these years. Writes Steve Hendricks in *Harper's*: 'There is evidence that the brain may even run more efficiently on ketones … this may account for the heightened sense of well-being and even euphoria that some fasters describe.'

Halfway into week two, I have gone from being barely able to lift a teaspoon to super-productive. I throw myself into job-hunting (I need to make some money to buy the food I will be eventually eating again), I write stories, I answer emails. I even feel strong enough to make plans to meet a friend in a restaurant. I can join in and have black tea! I can have water!

I'm as giddy as a gelding, arriving an hour early because I'm so excited to be out of the house. 'I was an hour early,' I tell my friend Lee at the sushi restaurant where I will watch her eat. 'I was so excited to see you, I got here an hour early – also I had nothing else to do!' Lee looks slightly worried, but compliments me on my weird wrinkle-free skin.

I am reminded of all those new mums I would meet who'd drink the house sparkling too fast or talk a million miles a minute – or just be way too excited to be in a fairly middling Thai restaurant. *It's just Thai, dude*, I would think. *Anyone would think you'd never been out, that you just spend all your time sitting indoors, at home* … Yeah, that. Now I am just like them, like a can of Coke that has been shaken up and opened, exploding everywhere. Out in the world, I am all nerves and excitement, clutching my friends with joy, like we've been separated for years. It is just a normal week for them, but I feel as if a death had occurred, and that death had been my own.

It's now day twelve and I've lost 8.3 kilograms. The mental alertness is still there and I proofread my novel. I am also writing again, covering everything from the abolition of the death penalty in South-East Asia to good places to eat in New Orleans. Smells and sights of food are fine. I sit at a cafe and drink a green tea and read the paper, without so much as a second glance (well, maybe a quick second glance) at the tray of pastries cooling nearby. That vicious hunger has gone. Maybe I could go on not eating forever … like a Breatharian! (At this point of the fast I feel a kinship with the much-maligned Breatharians.)

Then things shift again, as I'm learning they always do. By day thirteen I am starving. At night, I weep from hunger.

On the fourteenth day, I fall asleep in the afternoon – this sleep long, deep and peaceful – heavy with the sensation of swimming underwater without needing oxygen. It's like something from *The Tempest*:

> *Full fathom five thy father lies;*
> *Of his bones are coral made;*
> *Those are pearls that were his eyes:*
> *Nothing of him that doth fade,*
> *But doth suffer a sea-change*
> *Into something rich and strange.*

I too am suffering a sea change, into something rich and strange. It's all going on inside and I can only guess at what is happening at this subterranean level. As my symptoms morph, yet again, I wonder what level of the detox this is, what wave of cleaning is going on inside me.

By this time the cleaning guys must be wearing the hazard suits. It must be like Fukushima down there, where the nuclear stuff lies buried. The deep clean. But it's almost over. Almost. Soon I will be able to eat half a cucumber.

Half a cucumber! Half a cucumber! I'm so excited I shake off a lively, cinematic dream and get up early on the morning of day fifteen. My excitement levels are matching those of a six-year-old believer on Christmas morning. Today is the day! Today is the day! Breakfast. Break fast. Break. Fast. I take my monk's brew – black tea with a dollop of honey, then the foul herbs, heated up in a pan of water. Then I will (slowly) walk to the shops – a walk I have already done so many times in my head. I'm going to the fruit shop on Bondi Road, the expensive one I always complain about. Well, not any more! I'm going there, and I'm going to bury my head in a box of cucumbers, inhale deeply, with my extra-sensitive, heightened powers of smell, and select the cucumber that has the freshest, lightest, brightest smell. And then I'll eat it!

Breaking the fast correctly – and avoiding refeeding syndrome – is one of the most important ways to prevent any negative consequences. As well as slowing down enzyme production – because you're not digesting – when you eat again, you risk flooding your body with insulin as you shift suddenly from ketosis (fat-adapted metabolism) to carbohydrate-based foods. This process relies on nutrients that have been severely depleted during a fast: phosphate, potassium, magnesium and several vitamins, especially thiamine (vitamin B1). According to *Harper's*, 'Suddenly needing a lot of them leads to serious acute deficiencies, causing heart failure, hypotension, and sudden death.'

Sudden death.

So I eat the cucumber. First I wash it and peel it and cut it into long slices like fat, pale ribbons, then I lay the ribbons on a plate and go into the sunroom. The sun streams in, making the cucumber look jewelled, the pearl-coloured tiny beads or seeds – whatever they are – a miracle of design. The seeds (those jewels) rest in the whitish, firm flesh of the cucumber. If I wasn't so hungry, I could stare at it all day.

The cucumber was chosen to break the fast because it is – of all the things I could be sticking in my clean-as-a-whistle gut – the least likely to cause sudden death. No strong taste, smell, flavour – it is mostly water and fibre. Yet it is snappy and crunchy enough to provide some work for my teeth, to get them chewing again.

It is, I admit, not the stuff my food dreams are made of. I want something hot, deep-fried and oozing cheese. But, for now, it will do.

I have lasted the full fourteen days, which I am proud of – but I'm not out of the woods. I'm now entering phase two of the detox – in many ways more perilous than the first fourteen days. I have to stick to a very rigid eating plan of half a cucumber (all I am allowed for the day) plus the dreaded herbs, before moving on to 50 grams of poached chicken the next day, and one egg the day after.

Part of the appeal – if you can call it that – of fasting or restrictive diets is the notion that you can reset your tastebuds. It's like a hard restart or a system upgrade on your computer. You switch it off and the buggy bits – the bits that crave salt and grease and sugar – can be expelled, and in their place your body will crave salads, vegetables and gallons of water. Willpower isn't necessary when this happens. You just follow your cravings, and they will lead you to the organic vegetable aisle. The marketing person for the fasting clinic told me via email that the detox would reboot my system, that I would crave healthy food. It happened to her. But for me, it does not come to pass.

I crave all sorts of rubbish – mostly deep-fried, salty fast food like chicken wings. Yet my sense of portion size is radically reset, as is my attitude to alcohol. In the later stages of the fast I attend parties where I neither eat nor drink, and observe, not without some horror (did I used to be like that?), the way people would deteriorate over the course of a night. They would start off okay, then after an hour or two of drinking would stand too close to me, repeating the same story and spitting (did I used to spit?). Early in the night, I am so careful around the hors d'oeuvres ('Oh, none for me, thanks'), while they prowl like provo gangs around the perimeter of the party, looking for something – anything – to eat.

I don't walk around feeling superior to people when I'm on the fast, but I am full of wonder that people can eat *so much*. As my body is using its own fat (and muscle and bone) for fuel, and I am living off liquid herbs, anything more than a couple of small meals a day, with teeny-tiny portions of protein, carbs and vegetables, seems lavish – gluttonous, even. When I begin eating again, my portion sizes are so small and delicate that friends start

Instagramming them – incredulous that anyone would eat so little. 'Normal' meals are placed beside them for scale. But when you've been subsisting on liquid herbs then cucumber for weeks, what a feast it is to have one green bean (a longish one) and piece of fish that's roughly half the size of a credit card. My stomach has shrunk. I savour each flake.

As for alcohol, when I reintroduce it, I am shocked at how only one or two drinks gives me the world's worst hangover the following day. Two glasses of wine are debilitating. My clean body freaks the fuck out when it has to process the sugar, the alcohol and the chemicals. I ponder the nature of tolerance. My toxic body could cope so much better with lashings of alcohol and dirty foods. It soldiered on regardless. But after the fast I'm as sensitive as a poet. Is this what happens when you get clean? You become delicate?

The thing that drove me to the fast in the first place was not a sensitivity (the sort of sensitivity that leads others to complain of gluten intolerance or bloating or eczema) but its opposite – a sort of coarsening. My body was not a temple, it was a stockyard, where dirty animals passed through, where there was some horsetrading; it was busy and noisy and full of action. Stockyards are dynamic places, and useful things happen there. But they're far from the idea of the temple – and they're certainly not clean.

By day seventeen the allure of the cucumber is starting to wear thin. And I'm over the samey-ness of the herbs and the daily visits and weigh-ins at the fasting clinic. But energy continues to return to my body. Today I go to the beach for a run. When I sweat, there is curiously no odour. My tears no longer smell bad. The thick coating of ... something ... is disappearing from my tongue and in its place is this healthy pink thing that just longs to taste something.

I feel physically and mentally great. But the one thing that is missing is spiritual enlightenment. During the fast, there are no hallucinations or visions, no sense of oneness with the universe. If anything, the fast makes me feel separate and apart from the collective. I'm self-absorbed, and hyper-focused on my body and its processes. Such narcissism is surely the enemy of any sort of spiritual experience.

In the second stage of the fast I'll be attending a retreat where I'll be required to meditate for many hours a day, and I'm hoping that the discipline instilled by the fast will carry over to meditation. But that is a matter of tools and technique – none of the big, roaring, awesome, get-close-to-your-god stuff has occurred during the period of my starvation, and I sense none will occur in the fast's later stages.

On day twenty, I hit the closest point to giving up on the whole detox. It's the chest pains again. They wake me at 4am and I stay up until dawn, like I am standing vigil over a patient but the patient is me. I ring my editor, the one who gave me the assignment in the first place, and tell her that I'm worried about the side effects, that it feels like I'm having a heart attack, and that I'm scared. She takes me off the story immediately and urges me to see my doctor.

My doctor can't find anything wrong with my heart but books me in for a mammogram and an ECG, which sends me into an anxious spiral: breast cancer? A heart attack? What? All I wanted was to detox my life. My GP is more sanguine. He says fasting has been around forever and human beings are quite good at it, due to long periods of not catching things in the wilderness.

I do not feel so relaxed. I say sotto voce to my doctor, 'I've cheated.' I tell him about the hummus on New Year's Eve and the two grains of rice with Chris, and some of Jemma's breakfast. My doctor is very pleased. 'I'm glad,' he says. 'I'd worry what sort of person you are if you didn't cheat.'

Long after the fast, I speak to Amanda Salis about this second incident of alarming chest pains. She is blunt: 'It sounds dangerous to me. You felt like you were having a heart attack. Is that related to getting rid of toxins? If you deprive yourself of sufficient food for long enough, it will kill you.'

My body was eating its own muscle. Possibly the heart muscle. I was almost having a heart attack. Twice.

**

I am waiting for the results of my breast scan. What if I have cancer? I need to speak to someone who is not Dr Liu, my GP or my editor. At a barbecue in Melbourne before I commence the fast, a friend's brother told me about his colleague. Heather had done Dr Liu's detox and it changed her life. Heather had been a salt-of-the-earth broad of the old school, always getting drunk at the races, falling out of moving trams and getting into fights in the queue at McDonald's at 3am. Now she was skinny and well behaved. She became a Dr Liu convert and, in a way, a model of how I wanted my new self to be.

He put me on speaker and I chatted to Heather, who reassured me that even though it was the hardest thing she'd ever done, the fast was definitely worth it. Heather gave me her number and at least three email addresses. She told me the fast is so difficult that I'll need a mentor. She would be that mentor for me. She said, 'I'll be there for you. Just call. Anytime.'

I've contacted Heather every couple of days since I started the fast with a variety of fake-casual messages: 'Yo, what's up, bro, I'm just starvin' – I mean CHILLIN' – in da house …'

Now my messages are a lot less casual – it's like the narrative arc of Eminem's song 'Stan'.

'Hey, ring me back. Right now. Please. I think I am having a heart attack.'

'Hey, where are you? It's me, again. You said I could call you day and night. Well, I am calling you and you are, you are …'

You are, where?

I never get a reply from Heather. During this detox, it becomes clear that there's one thing I need that I don't have – a friend. This is rough stuff to do on your own. Later, after my article comes out, people find me – people who are in days five or more of the detox. They are suffering and reaching out. They want to know – does it work? Will I be okay? I answer quickly and soothe them like I wanted to be soothed: *Everything will be all right. It will all be okay.*

My editor keeps emailing and asking if I am eating again, telling me that everyone in the office is worried about my wellbeing. When I went to see her at Fairfax HQ a few days ago, everyone was shocked at how different I looked. One editor even thought that I'd shrunk in terms of *height*. The fast had made me shorter! (Amanda Salis later tells me that a detox this extreme can result in the body eating bone in order to stay alive, leading to osteoporotic fractures of the vertebrae that can shorten you by several centimetres – so maybe I was actually getting shorter.)

My friend Viv, who used to be a nurse, comes with me to get my chest pain test results. I am shaking in the passenger seat of her car. She opens the envelopes and reads the X-rays. The cancer tests come back negative. The ECG is normal – and the weight keeps dropping off.

I continue to see Dr Liu, who tells me 'progress will be slow' but he will get me down to my 'natural body shape'. Even though I only see him a few times during the course of my treatment, I know he is monitoring my daily weigh-ins and I obscurely want to please him. I'm not doing it for me; I'm doing it for Dr Liu. Months after the fast proper finishes my diary is full of things like 'I went out and had some chicken pho. Cannot believe it. What would Dr Liu think?' *What would Dr Liu think* – I wondered this all through the first six months of that year, whenever anything plea-surable passed my lips. But perhaps we need an authority figure when we do something as grave, risky and difficult as not eating. In order to actually persevere we must create either a bogeyman or a father figure – someone stern, whom we fear if we go off course, someone we want to please, whose approval we crave.

I leave Sydney and go stay with my parents in the coastal hamlet of Port Fairy. Each night they cook amazing food, which they don't serve me. I am sulky and depressed and heat up the packets of herbs, which I drink away from everyone like the special case I've become.

It's a warm summer and they are entertaining a lot – eggs and bacon in the morning, long, bracing walks along the beach fol-lowed by lattes in sidewalk cafes, a drinks cabinet on wheels on the porch and jugs of Pimm's in the afternoon, cheese and biscuits, the smell of barbecue and the beads of sweat running down the neck of a beer.

Why is it that you only recognise paradise once it's been lost?

But in high cupboards are my old clothes, and there is an amazing satisfaction to slipping on a pair of pants last worn twenty years ago and having them zip right up to the top instead of giving up halfway there. People stop me in the street, to exclaim over not my weight loss but the weird anti-ageing thing I have going on. It's nothing like the look of people who've had surgery and emerge – suddenly, somewhat horrifically – looking 'refreshed', but rather a strange face that belongs to someone ten, twenty years younger than me.

So is fasting a bad or a good thing?

It depends who you ask. There is an enormous gap between what the wellness 'experts' say and what mainstream medicine says about fasting. The former say it's the cure; the latter – crudely speaking – says it's the disease. Moderate forms of fasting such as the 5:2 diet have been approved by many in the medical profession, but a long and extreme fast, such as the one I undertook, is pre-modern, frontier medicine, left over from a time of leeches, blood-letting and purging. Now and then, though, studies emerge on the effects of fasting on hypertension, or the immune cell response in certain cancers, or on epilepsy. And the results (remember this is no drugs, no treatment, just the patient not eating) can seem to verge on miraculous. But we're a long way away from consensus within the scientific community, and as for consensus between medical and wellness experts – they're not even speaking the same language.

But I am interested in the hunger cure for illnesses. Twain talked of starving out a cold or flu, of starvation being the best medicine. And sometimes this has proven to be the case, despite a long fast being seen more as alternative as opposed to mainstream medicine. US studies in the 1930s showed that fasting followed by a high-fat diet were successful in reducing epileptic seizures, and prior to the manufacture of insulin, fasting was showing signs in early trials of success in reducing symptoms for childhood diabetes.

In a more recent trial, Valter Longo, Professor of Gerontology and the Biological Sciences at the USC Davis School of Gerontology and director of the USC Longevity Institute, is studying how fasting benefits the immune system – with a particular focus on people with cancer who are undergoing chemotherapy treatment. His studies with mice found a couple of things: the efficacy of chemo was improved with periods of long fasting. Twenty per cent of mice in which the cancer had fully spread, and 40 per cent with a more limited spread, were completely cured after fasting in conjunction with chemotherapy. All the mice who just had chemotherapy died.

In 2014 Longo told the *Daily Telegraph* that when you starve, 'The system tries to save energy, and one of the things it can do to save energy is to recycle a lot of the immune cells that are not needed, especially those that may be damaged ... Everything [is getting] a little younger and it goes back to working much better.'

A long fast means the body uses its stores of glucose, fat and ketones and also breaks down a significant portion of white blood cells, which trigger stem cell–based regeneration of new immune system cells, according to Longo's research, published in the journal *Cell*.

Longo's research is ongoing; human trials are underway.

As for my own experience, I can say this: there was a terrible feeling in my body in America. It was the feeling of excess – too much drinking, smoking, drugs, bad food, not doing enough exercise and not sleeping properly. I remember a cab speeding to the airport in

Las Vegas, and me saying, 'Step on it, step on it' – another doomed attempt to catch a plane after a night on the Strip that ended in a desert dawn. The cab driver looked at me in the rear-view mirror and said softly, not unkindly, 'You know, honey, this wouldn't happen if you took better care of yourself.'

Fast-forward to December and it's cold. I am in New York. I could feel myself getting sick, and as I tried to coax the feral cat I was minding in the windowless 20-square-foot apartment in Manhattan, to play with her toy made out of an empty tissue box, I felt about ninety years old. Everything ached. It felt like the opposite of vitality. Fasting – in the end – brought that vitality back.

Around the time I start my fast, food Instagrammers are in the ascendancy. The ones I follow, mostly young women on the hashtag #cleaneating, are very thin, white and wealthy. They holiday in places like St Barthélemy and Ibiza. They don't eat sugar, gluten or dairy, yet despite their asceticism they somehow manage to style a chia-seed pudding into something moreish and desirable. In some shots the Instagrammers are doing yoga headstands, and in others they are on yachts. Sometimes they post memes that in my weakened state I find encouraging. 'Do not reward yourself with food, you are not a dog,' says one that I stare at for a long time, the screen glowing in my dark bedroom.

But a counter-trend is emerging. All over the country, the hippest new restaurants are selling dude food – burgers, fried chicken, ribs, mac and cheese, schnitzels and fries. It's suddenly cool (and expensive) to dine at an indie version of KFC. The reviews talk lovingly of fryers imported from Tennessee and different types of lard, recommending the best beers to wash it all down with. This is dirty food – my sort of food. There are also monster milkshakes in mason jars filled with sugary milk, syrup and chocolate bars and jammed with doughnuts. People are queuing up to get in. If you want to eat out you have a choice of some expensive pressed-juice and salad bar or some place that sells expensive, high-calorie, deep-South Americana fare. Where are all the *normal* cafes? It's as if society itself has a form of disordered eating.

In the old, serious newspapers, pages three and five – and sometimes page one – are giving over, breathlessly, to a new food trend. These food trends often seem to be verging on parody, as if the chefs and the baristas and the editors have got together and tried to top each other in decadence or frivolity, collaborating to see how far we the readers can be pushed into buying it.

We're all foodies now, or aspire to be. The language of restaurants (what's in, what's good, what's new, what's opening and shutting), ingredients, chefs, new methods of food preparation, of recently discovered superfoods, has become a currency of sorts. In this world, it's no surprise Australia's fastest-growing media success story is *Broadsheet*, which each week publishes news of the hottest restaurant openings, lovingly detailing the ancestry of the coffee beans or the revival of the early-twentieth-century butter churn. When *Broadsheet* writes about a new restaurant opening in Melbourne or Sydney, the next day there are queues around the block. Restaurateurs talk about this effect. They call it being 'broadshat'.

In 2015 I reviewed restaurants for *Guardian Australia* – which was great, except I could never really shake the feeling that I was engaged in the promotion of a lifestyle that seemed overly lavish, wasteful and frivolous: a symptom of a society that has become too wealthy for its own good. I like good food. I love restaurants. But hitting all the hatted restaurants week in, week out – it was impossible to ignore the decadence. More than one person in the industry told me these years felt like Rome before the fall.

There were the elaborate menus with ten or more tiny dishes, each containing dozens of ingredients – with some of these ingredients being so rare that in order to procure them, one must forage in a remote forest in central America. The rare ingredients are then flown halfway around the world to sit on top of your parfait, and consumed without a moment's thought for the energy expended on getting them from 'paddock to plate'.

There were the juice sommeliers who ran through the 'juice matching options' at only $140 extra a head, if you weren't drinking alcohol.

And the no-cancellation policies.

There were the amuses-bouche, always, and the little things that came 'compliments of the chef'.

There were the plates designed by a former investment banker turned potter in Northcote and fired in a kiln imported from Galway.

There was the feeling, around three-quarters into the meal, that you weren't going to last, that there was too much food, and you would have to – just like the Romans – go and purge your stomach in order to make room for dessert.

There were priceless wine cellars and the months-long waitlist for a $600-a-head dinner at Noma, the ballot for a degustation at the Fat Duck.

There was the waiter crouching at your table, telling you in loving detail about the farm in Gippsland where your lamb was raised.

There were the people Instagramming their food at the next table. There were the restaurants that were no longer really restaurants – instead they were tourist destinations and forms of social media currency – and anyway getting a reservation was impossible.

One night, after reviewing three restaurants in Melbourne – including the grim, multi-course Zumbo dessert degustation, I got into a taxi and my pants split.

It was time to start writing about something else.

Australians throw out $8 billion of edible food every year – much of which is fruit and vegetables. Our good intentions take us through the supermarket check-out but much of the greenery dies on the fridge shelf, along with our healthful aspirations.

It's not packets of chips or chocolate bars that end up in the bin – Australians eat 32 kilograms of chocolate per person, per year. Corporations have spent billions on research and development to find our sweet spots when it comes to junk food – the perfect balance of sugar, fat and salt that goes into a corn chip, for example, or a chocolate bar.

These processed foods are being marketed to us with billion-dollar budgets. And they are cheap – they don't cost much, compared with, say, grain-fed beef or organic kale. The bind? We buy the processed foods that are sold so aggressively to us, but then we are made to feel shame when we eat them – or eat too much of them.

I'm sure I'm not the only person to run on this particular treadmill (this is purely a metaphor; there are no literal treadmills here) – excess followed by guilt followed by self-imposed false deprivation. The weekend of pizza and beers, chips and pinot gris, followed by regret and the Monday-morning diet. The hedonism followed by the asceticism.

It's not a new thing, this all-then-nothing approach. Fasting occurred naturally in primitive man after feasting – a necessity due to uncertain food supply. Then it became incorporated into ritual (the Romans with their feasts and purging) and religion.

Now in a post-religious, post-ritual age, many of us rely on a different sort of calendar. It's the party calendar – the Christmas season that kicks off early in November around the time of the Melbourne Cup and ends with Australia Day. It's the long, hot hedonistic time of year when we go out every night, drink and eat too much, and say, 'What the hell,' or simply just, 'Hello,' to the proffered profiterole or line of coke or cigarette or bottle of champagne. Hey, it's summer. Next please, yes thanks and more, more, more. Maybe it's greed, maybe it's habit, maybe it's because everyone else is doing it – but the brakes are off for three months.

Then February, and the detox cycle begins. We crave to be clean. The market is ready – as the market always is. There are detox spas here and in South-East Asia, where they'll not feed you for a hefty fee. There are all the gyms with their *New Year, New You!* advertising and the boot camps and the personal trainers and the protein shakes and pharmacy detox kits. There are diet books and eating plans and internet forums with programs by Michelle Bridges (mindset), Sarah Wilson (no sugar) and Pete Evans (Paleo). Some of these programs are a neat twelve weeks, unintended echoes perhaps of the Twelve-Step Alcoholics Anonymous program.

They're all here to help us, to wish us well – all the Petes and Sarahs and Michelles – waiting at the end of the party, to scoop us up and promise us that if we do as they say, follow their program and go without (for fuck's sake, just this once!) then equilibrium and vitality will be restored.

In all this there is the idea of reversal and redemption. Here we are again (and again and again), lashed to the pendulum of excess and starvation. Why are there so many of us who can't live in the middle? What is it that we're really looking for?

Between the hedonism and the clean eating falls the shadow. The detox cycle has its own attendant emotions – mostly guilt, sometimes self-disgust, recriminations and reprisals, fear of change rooms, avoidance of mirrors and certain close-fitting clothes – yet there is also the promise and hope of a new year and new diet that some friend or other has tried that *really worked*. I experienced all those ugly emotions towards the end of my time in New York. I hated being in my skin and in my clothes (I also hated being out of my clothes) but there it was on the horizon – the thing that kept me from total self-loathing and despair. As regularly as February rolls around, there is this promise – I'm going to detox.

About fifteen years ago, before clean eating and online wellness programs and Instagram, I read a book called *The Clothesline Diet* that stayed with me. It wasn't the diet itself that I cared about, but the stories of the women in it. They walked around their backyard clotheslines to lose weight. These were women in towns without gyms, or women with young children who couldn't leave the house, or women without much money, or women too embarrassed about their size to exercise in public. It was a working-class book, earthy – not aspirational. The women were the carers of young children, of ageing parents, of everyone but themselves. (Caitlin Moran wrote memorably in her book *How to Be a Woman*, 'Overeating is the addiction of choice of carers, and that's why it's come to be regarded as the lowest-ranking of all the addictions. It's a way of screwing yourself up whilst still remaining fully functional, because you have to.')

The first-person accounts of how the women had put on weight were gripping: all the visits to the drive-thru on the way to school pick-up and the burgers crammed in the mouth, engine idling in the parking lot. The eating late at night. The secret eating. The two dinners – one with the kids and one with the husband. The bag of lollies or chips in front of the TV after the kids are in bed. The biscuits with the cup of tea – and before you know it the pack is gone. Such small sins, followed by self-loathing.

The book sparked a sense that in the future (which has now well and truly arrived), the struggles, the tests and triumphs we would face would be with ourselves. Our own bodies would be the sites of battle. And so it came to pass in shows such as *The Biggest Loser*. Narrative was an important part of it – how we got here, how we let ourselves go and how we're going to take charge again. How we were going to become clean.

In this age of extreme narcissism, our victories are not against an outside force or an injustice, they are not *public* or *social* victories but small, private things: triumphs over our own bodies' appetites and our own weak characters.

I wonder how many other people out there are starving themselves. I suspect my fellow fasters are everywhere – I see them on the magazines on all the newsagent shelves. How else would some-one lose five kilograms in a week to get a *bikini-ready* body?

But pick up the magazine a few months later, and they're back to what they were – body-shamed with a red circle on their thighs. It's the new scarlet letter.

The wellness industry and the diet industry are distinct but over-lapping beasts. To diet is to follow a regime, in the relative short term, in order to achieve a weight-loss goal. The wellness indus-try talks about nutrition as something that you internalise and just *do*. It has no end; in fact, weight loss is rarely mentioned. Overall health is the marker of success. The word 'clean' is used instead of 'thin'. You are judged not just on weight but also on tone and glow. There is a moral component too: is the food locally grown and sourced? Is it organic? Is it cruelty free? Is it grain- or grass-fed? Has it been processed using industrial farming methods? Did its planting displace indigenous crops?

Wellness – on Instagram at least – is all about signalling. Consumption is conspicuous. How you eat is a dog whistle of sorts, a sign that you are a certain sort of person, with particular values, level of intelligence and spending power. The cleaner you eat, the higher you are up the hierarchy. As Hayley Phelan writes in *Vogue*, wellness is 'the new luxury status symbol ... If five years ago it was a Céline bag, today's ultimate status symbol might just be a SoulCycle hoodie and a green juice'. And Hadley Freeman in the *Guardian*: 'Ostentatiously ascetic good health is now a major fashion trend ... The pursuit of "wellness" hits that crucial point on the Venn diagram between aspiration, self-love and slimness.'

There is also a class aspect at play. If you are poor, you won't be paying forty dollars for that Himalayan pink salt.

It reminds me of being at a supermarket in Sydney with a friend's children. This friend eats really well, and is into organic produce. We were walking down the aisles behind a family that you could describe as obese. The mum was putting chips, chocolate and frozen foods in their trolley. The children I was with laughed and pointed, but didn't call the family 'fat', they called them 'fat and poor'.

**

N+1 editor Mark Greif writes, 'Having our food supply made simple, we devote ourselves to looking for ways to make it difficult.' Dieting, he says, with its 'weight-loss imperative, with its shadows of attractiveness and social distinction, and other fantasies of rarity, difficulty and expense, complicates the fairly mundane research consensus on improving health: eat moderately, move more.' He goes on:

> Frankly, I suspect that an ethics of living in a rich nation
> at the dawn of the 21st century involves not caring so
> much about your health, your diet, your exercise and
> your thrills. The meaningful time is now. We should be
> prepared to enjoy our good luck, and drop dead after a
> sufficient length of time – but ask, along the way, what we
> actually wish to do with our time.

Wellness is a treadmill, and sucks up so much time and money – isn't it worth pondering how much of it really helpful? At the Global Wellness Summit held in Austria in 2016, ten major wellness trends were identified. Among them was the optimistically titled 'From Superfood and Diet Trend Hysteria to Sane Eating'. According to materials released by the summit, 'The last few years have been marked by a near-hysterical obsession with the next superfood or diet trend. So much so that experts are suggesting that this age of diet-hopping and food puritanism may be a collective, global eating disorder.'

There is no better example of complication and food puritanism than 'clean eating', which is based on a fear on ingesting toxins and a fixation on the providence and 'purity' of foods. Clean eating has become the sort of gold standard of the eating world – and requires rigorous discipline and policing. You also need to have a fair amount of time and money to constantly eat clean. It's the sort of diet that you organise your life around. The madness of this is never remarked upon; indeed, this way of living is prized. Maybe it's our *collective, global eating disorder*.

In its extreme form, clean eating can tip over into 'orthorexia nervosa', a term coined in 1997 when Dr Steven Bratman detailed his eating regime: he wouldn't eat vegetables picked more than fifteen minutes earlier and chewed every mouthful fifty times. Bratman defined his condition as 'a pathological fixation on eating proper food' or a fixation on righteous eating.

Experts such as dietitian Tania Ferraretto say a modern obsession with clean eating is fuelling more cases of orthorexia nervosa. She told the ABC, 'People are getting their [dietary] information from lots of different sources, and most of these sources are actually very un-credible, and providing potentially dangerous information.' She says orthorexia often falls under the radar, because people who have it look healthy, when really they aren't.

On Instagram, the hashtag #cleaneating has more than 28 million posts.

Londoner Carrie Armstrong, thirty-five, became obsessed with 'clean' eating after she was struck down by a virus eight years ago. According to the *Guardian*, she was bed-bound and unable to lift her head off the pillow. Doctors said there was little more that medicine could do, so to speed up her natural recovery, she began researching alternative remedies and diets online.

'My first thought was no wonder I had got so sick because I'd been eating badly for years,' she says. 'But then I started reading about the transformative effects of giving up meat and sugar, then carbohydrates, and it went from there.' Armstrong went vegan then switched to raw veganism, renouncing all animal-based food products and anything that had been cooked. Over eighteen months she dropped from 70 to 40 kilograms, stopped menstruating, and became 'completely obsessed' with 'detoxing and cleansing'.

In August 2016 a Sydney woman was sentenced to fourteen months' jail, suspended, after she fasted while breastfeeding her child. She had been treating her son for severe eczema, first via a restrictive diet and then a fast, on recommendation by a naturopath. When the woman took her eight-month-old son to hospital in 2015, he was emaciated and severely dehydrated, had sunken eyes, dangerously low sodium levels and 'flexed hands and feet'. 'Had he not presented at hospital at that time, he would have died within days,' the magistrate Ian Guy said. The woman's family noticed the child's and her own weight loss and told her to stop the diet, but she did not. At one point, she modified the water-only rule by eating only watermelon for three days. (This is what I would call 'cheating' if I had done this on my fast.)

An evidence-based medicine specialist with Bond University, Professor Chris Del Mar, told the *Guardian* that the naturopathic industry was almost 'impossible' to regulate, given there were no restrictions on who could call themselves a naturopath.

He said the parents of a sick child seeing a naturopath might not realise illness was the effect of the treatment rather than a cause, and therefore might end up seeking further naturopathic treatment. This is the so-called healing crisis paradox.

S o how did I go off the detox? To paraphrase the character Mike in Hemingway's *The Sun Also Rises*: gradually then suddenly.

For around the first thirty days I followed the fast (almost) to the letter, but it was too restrictive to continue much longer than that. I did a fairly consistent but modified version until day eighty-three. By the end I felt and looked great – possibly the best I've ever looked. Plus I was full of energy and vigour. I lost about 12 kilograms, normalised my cholesterol and blood pressure levels and went off medication for these conditions.

But the discipline was not to last. I was the girl with the self-control and the delicate portions for around three months. I was the girl with the waistline she'd had when she was eighteen. I was the girl with the new, small clothes. Then things – well, they roared back to life. What pushed me back into my bad old pre-fast ways was the thing I had been really craving in all those summer months in Bondi – a job.

When you get serious about looking for a job, and then when you get a job, the thing you need the most is fuel. One bean, a piece of steamed fish half the size of an iPhone 5, half a cucumber, 50 grams of poached chicken – that shit won't even get you out the door.

It's all right lolling around in your disgusting bed all day, losing weight through your stinking breath, if you have nowhere else to be, nowhere to go, no job or boyfriend or family nearby. You can exist in a state of funky ketosis until you've burnt through your bones, the bedclothes and all that lies beneath.

But sooner or later you need to rejoin the world. My new job would take me back to Melbourne. All nerves and adrenalin, I rehearsed my lines at the airport on the way to the interview. *Maybe I'll be better able to focus if I have a coffee*, I thought. Then I realised I didn't need an excuse. There was no omniscient fasting god staring down at me; Dr Liu needn't know. If I wanted a coffee then I should have a coffee. I went to MoVida and ordered a flat white. When it came I dipped my head to it, like I was praying to a milky deity.

One coffee begets another. In Melbourne I had meetings, during which it's customary to take coffee. To drink herbal tea or water is to mark you out as a stranger in the city, a non-native – like not having a football team to barrack for.

Food came soon after the job. Then booze. I moved to a flat in St Kilda and started work in the city at 6am. Winter came early and there was comfort in the things that warmed you up: the tram coming on time in Bourke Street, a heated train carriage, a steaming plate of scrambled eggs from Self Preservation, the trays and trays and trays of coffees – the paper cups piling up on the news desk, people's names misspelt on the side. Leaves crunchy underfoot, the way your breath would cling to the air, and the sound, far away as you fast-walked down Grey Street, of the trams turning and gliding up Fitzroy Street. The soundtrack of that winter was Beck's *Morning Phase* – melancholy, melodious, a paean to endings.

It was the winter of the Negroni – the solid blocks of ice and the wedge of orange, the tart, sweet, spicy tang, like an older man's aftershave. It was also a good year for truffles. They came on everything – eggs, pizza, pasta, soups. I ate them all.

I'd forgotten the subtle differences between the two cities. I associated Sydney with wellness, and Melbourne with a more interior life. Even the yoga studios seemed darker – fewer pot plants and arch windows, and more womb-like, where the shavasana and the reverberations of a gong felt like they could go on forever.

Back in Melbourne, I became, again, thankful for food and booze. I was aware – and this was not a bad thing – how comforting it could be. Sometimes on a bad day, the thought of a tasty, hot meal was what got me through. And there's nothing, really, wrong with that.

Days toiling at the digital coalface of the news cycle (and what a cycle it was – ISIS and desert beheadings, the spread of Ebola, girls kidnapped by Boko Haram and Malaysia Airlines planes going missing and being shot down), relentless and without a sense of completion, it was coffee that kept me up and alcohol that brought me down. It was drinks in the laneway bars near the office where I got to know my colleagues. *The meaningful time is now.*

Luckily I didn't throw out my old 'fat' clothes; I eventually ended up at the weight I started. What goes down must come up. Several months after I stopped fasting and the weight returned, my blood pressure levels went back to a high reading and I returned to taking blood pressure medication. But something in me had shifted. I think it was the knowledge that if I really wanted to lose a lot of weight, I could do it. But I was making a choice – and that choice was one of drinking and eating what took my fancy. Of enjoying food, and making it central. Of not saying no to anything (within reason). At other times of my life I might not see food in this way, but at this time I did.

Dr Liu suggested I go on the full fast again – stop eating, and just start drinking the foul herbs, but my heart wasn't in it. I had been clean – achieved that almost miraculous, hard-fought place where it felt like every toxin harboured had exited my body. Getting to this level of clean was the wellness equivalent of Scientology's 'going clear' – the highest state of enlightenment you can achieve, a special place only a few can enter. But I didn't think I could do it again. The detox was a journey alone to a place where nothing grew, somewhere austere, with hard soil, and a beating, pitiless sky. I now understood why, in allegory, mystics and saints are always fasting in a desert. It's a hard, lonely place without the solace of distraction. But I had just been passing through. I did not want to go back.

LEAN

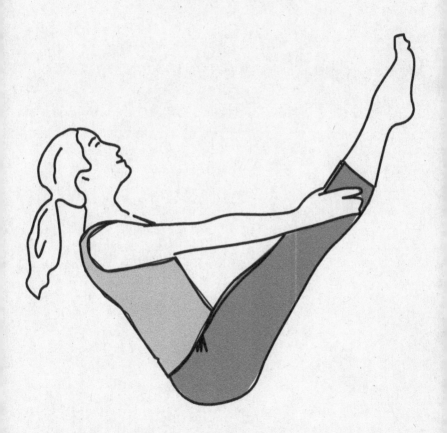

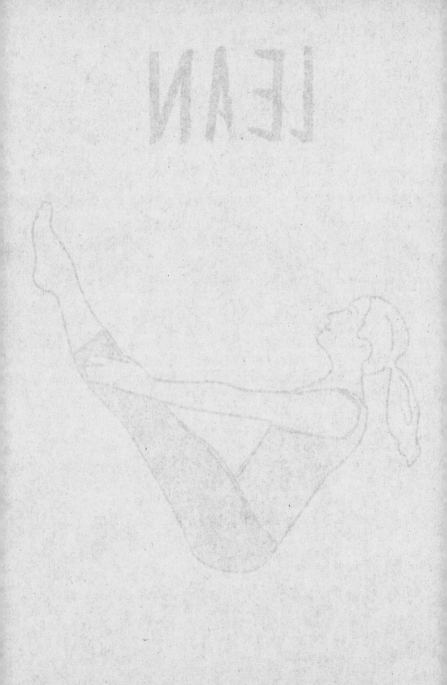

'm sitting in a hotel suite with expansive views of Sydney Harbour. In the room are two yoga instructors so vital and glowing that they seem burnished. They are literally sitting at the feet of Bikram Choudhury, founder of the yoga that bears his name.

I am there to interview Bikram because he is about to open his first yoga studio in Australia. In the 1970s he developed a new form of yoga that takes place in a room heated to almost 41 degrees with 40 per cent humidity. The heat is said to allow for deeper stretching and injury prevention. Classes run for ninety minutes and consist of a set series of twenty-six postures and two breathing exercises. They have become wildly successful – particularly with celebrities – and Bikram is earning a tonne of money from copyrighting and franchising this type of hot yoga all over the world. He is a fierce guardian of his brand and very litigious if he suspects you of ripping off any of his 'moves'.

A photographer and I had visited the studio earlier in the day. The room was boiling hot. It smelt like a mixture of ammonia and wet school uniform. It was wall-to-wall flesh, with most people wearing just inches of material – short shorts or bikini bottoms, tank tops or, for the men, nothing on top. Participants glistened, turned and baked like rotisserie chooks. The mirrors were steamed and sweating too, and made it look like there were hundreds of people in there – duplicates, triplicates – disciples in the tropics, performing an intricate choreography. The photographer moved around the edges, taking pictures and sweating heavily. I took notes, red-faced and uncomfortable. The atmosphere in the room was too close, too intense. Once we got the shots we needed, we left. And now in the hotel room, Bikram Choudhury, who is discussing plans to further franchise his yoga, looks me up and down.

'You,' he says. 'You need to do some Bikram. You are overweight.'

I am lost for words. He then goes on to describe some enormous woman – some morbidly obese giantess! – who had done his brand of yoga and ended up resembling the pair of lithe yoga instructors seated at his feet. They seem neither young nor old, but look very tanned, taut, serene and slightly vacant – like you'd imagine anyone would look after spending a lot of time exercising in a very hot room.

'Do my yoga,' he says, 'and you could look like them.'

But … but … What if I don't want to look like them? What if I want to look like *me*?

I leave the interview fuming and begin a determined sanction against all things Bikram.

'Fuck you, Bikram,' I mutter under my breath as I pass his studio, with its steamed-up windows and vile stench.

After my gentle, non-heated, mantra-chanting, omm-omming, stretchy, non-Bikram yoga I go to a cafe and drink chai with people from my class and we pay out on Bikram.

'It's, like, totally commercial. Yoga fast food. He's trademarked it. You need to, like, train in LA or something before you can teach it. Celebrities do it.'

The yoga people screw up their noses at the mention of LA and the celebrities.

'I've met Bikram, you know, the guy who invented the yoga. He was staying in a five-star hotel on the harbour.'

The yoga people screw up their noses at the mention of the five-star hotel and the harbour views. I don't tell them that Bikram called me fat.

The trade sanctions go on for years. I get a personal trainer. I do Pilates. I decide to learn how to run, but – like an elderly person – I am plagued by a dodgy hip. I swim. I start Zumba. I do Step. I get injured again and have long periods of inactivity followed by short bursts of frantic exercise. I gym-hop. I negotiate direct debits. I negotiate to rescind my direct debits. Occasionally I meet someone who does Bikram and I recall my meeting with its founder with the waning ferocity of a crotchety veteran of some long-ago war.

I start to wonder, *Bikram and me – what was it that we were fighting about?* Maybe in his brutal way, he was trying to help me. Maybe he really cared about my health. And anyway, hadn't I interviewed him with a hangover? Maybe he was trying to be kind. Maybe he had my best interests at heart. Maybe it's time to lay down my weapons.

So, six years after my first encounter with Bikram, I walk into one of his studios, a place up some stairs on Johnston Street in Fitzroy, Melbourne, and take my first class.

I imagine this is what being born feels like. My skin is a livid pink, I am covered in a fluid that has a primal, vaguely amniotic quality and I am lying on my back in an upturned fetal position. The urge to cry out for my mother is strong.

As often happens when you try something new and strange, time takes on a non-linear quality. It lengthens. There's an excess of it, like a ball of wool that unravels and spools from your hands. *Is it an hour into my first Bikram class or has it been ten? When will it end?* I wonder with a sort of detached desperation. I have been told no matter what happens in this first class, I must stay in the room. The room is heated to almost 41 degrees. I hate the heat but I must take the heat.

There are maybe thirty people in the studio, all staring fixedly at themselves in the front mirror. They are mostly nearly naked. Almost all are tattooed. All – at the one-hour mark – are covered in the slime-like sweat.

I watch it bead and drip from parts of my body that I never thought could produce sweat, let alone in such vast quantities. Out it comes from my calves, the soles of my feet, the inside of my arms, my hair, my earlobes. When I do an inverted pose, the sweat runs into my mouth and I accidentally swallow it. It has the consistency of olive oil and tastes – unsurprisingly – of sweat.

Other people's sweat flicks around the room in drips and spurts. The guy on the mat in front of me leans down to do eagle pose and drips his foot-sweat into my face; my next-door neighbour's ponytail flicks a stream of sweat onto my mat, like a horse after a race.

The instructors are miked and stand up the front. This could be a military drill. 'Legs should be like concrete, steel ... one piece, unbroken.' Many of the postures rely on constrictions, where you 'choke your throat', then release, gasping for air in the heat.

Afterwards in the change rooms hardly anyone speaks and no one makes eye contact – like a bad one-night stand where you finish up quickly and bolt for the door. But after that first class, something incredible happens to me. Euphoria. And it's not just the usual endorphin rush, but something akin to a drug high. Everything is as it should be. Everything is beautiful. My mind is calm and my body feels twisted, rinsed and lengthened from the inside out.

I start going two, three, five times a week – as often as I can, just so I can experience that thing on the mat: being drenched in sweat, being born again – the thing that cults or religion or exercise promise and this so viscerally delivers. Each time feels like the first time.

Sometimes in class people cry, or are sick. They try to leave, or they stand up and look disorientated before flopping onto their backs in a recovery posture.

By the end of the first, intensive month, I'm losing weight and feeling strong and everything – particularly my limbs – feels and looks elongated.

I also feel like the yoga is tuning me in to a higher frequency. I start receiving quasi-spiritual, career-orientated messages when I come out of tough poses. It's like Bikram himself is speaking to me in his gruff, mean way about what I should do with my life. In one class I receive what can only be described as a flood of insight while doing a super-intense backbend. While coming out of the camel pose a very authoritative voice from within commands that I must return to the law and retrain to be a barrister. It is very specific. In the week after the class I buy the textbooks, sign up for the exam to do the Readers' Course, find a barrister to read with and an office to squat in, and start preparing for the exam. In other words, I up-end my life because of an insight I had in a yoga class. I study civil procedure, evidence law and criminal law for six months before a senior barrister takes me out to lunch to interrogate me on how much I *really* want to be a barrister. 'What made you decide to change careers?' he asks. I do not tell him it was Bikram.

In the end neither the study nor the Bikram stick. After six months I move house, and with the studio an extra two tram rides away, I stop going. Then I move to New York and throw in the study. Nothing I read seems to be retained in my brain.

After I leave Bikram, I remember only the annoying things: my yoga clothes wet and heavy in the bottom of a sports bag, the way they smelt, even after I'd washed them. The way *I* smelt, even after a shower. The way the studio smelt, and the way its sodden carpet (floorboards were too risky – you could have an accident slipping on the sweat) would always smell of vomit, no matter how much they'd been cleaned. All this gives me reason not to take up Bikram again.

I don't miss it.

But my body never forgets it. Doing something every day – even for just one month – imprints on my muscles and their memory. Even now, hearing someone say the words 'standing bow pulling pose' makes my body instinctively want to bend deeply at the hips. I can do things, move in a certain way, bend and stretch in a way – right back my knees, head to heels – that looks almost like an angel has come into my body and gently removed my ribs. All because of Bikram.

Yoga – the activity that is the pathway for many people into the wellness industrial complex – has entered the mainstream in the last decade. Just walk through any city or suburban main street and look up. There's sure to be a yoga studio up a narrow flight of stairs. Sometimes it's Bikram, sometimes a generic hot yoga, or hip-hop yoga or hatha. An Ibis market research report from 2015 on the industry in Australia noted the sharp growth of yoga in the last decade. It has now become Australia's fastest-growing sports, its popularity doubling in the past eight years.

Where I live, in Bondi, there are now a dozen studios, but I remember when there used to be just one – Dharma Shala in North Bondi. The scent of incense and the ocean hung heavy, along with the sweaty, rubbery odour of old yoga mats. Ragged Tibetan prayer flags flapped out the front. Mist drifted in the air and on cold, still nights you could hear the waves crashing against the cliffs at Ben Buckler Point. Young people weren't represented so much – there were more older men in the class: rich hippies with bad backs who'd spent formative years in India or Bali. They were men of inscrutable spirituality who didn't come in pony-tailed packs but alone – snakes shedding their skin weekly, doing the moves with a sort of vacillating coiled, uncoiled, coiled intensity, like they'd been doing it forever, like they'd been doing it all their past lives. The practice felt like something deeply private that you just happened to do in public. And this public space was muted: the blinds were drawn, the lights dim, the sounds of the waves high and close, and the room had a hushed, cathedral-like atmosphere of people praying alone. I always felt stretched out and revived after a class. Good was being done, somehow, somewhere in my body. And so I kept going.

Later a really cool organic cafe opened next door, and a different, younger crowd started attending classes – one more conspicuously healthy, cliquey, better dressed and voluble. This was the emergence of a new tribe – a curious blend of hippy and yuppy, a sort of wellness version of the bourgeois bohemians. They saw yoga not just as an exercise class but as a lifestyle. They talked about yoga retreats in Costa Rica over chai tea and green juice, their yoga mats lined, bright and upright, like umbrellas against the door.

This was before the Instagrammers and the #cleaneaters, but this group was a bridge between back then and now, a sort of bellwether for wellness – a wellwether, if you like – that became a model for not just how we should look, and what we should wear, but the rest of it: what we should do and how we should *be*.

Now the tribe has grown further and the aesthetic that used to belong to just one corner of North Bondi and the wellness capitals of LA, New York, Costa Rica, Ubud and San Francisco has spread out to the suburbs, towns and regions.

It's activewear as a default uniform, tattoos in Sanskrit or inked lines from Rumi or Beckett ('Fail again, fail better'), cold-pressed juice bars, salad outlets, breakfast bowls and activated almonds. It's mindfulness apps, #cleaneating, yoga retreats, yoga teacher training, the fusion between yoga and surfing culture, the Buddha statue in the garden of the glass-and-steel beach house, the $120 yoga mats, the resale market on second-hand Lululemon leggings, the alkalised water, the coconut water, the coconut.

Roy Morgan Research from 2016 said one in ten Australians aged fourteen and over now do yoga, up from one in twenty in 2008 when aerobics ruled.

Today, more than twice as many people do yoga than aerobics. Yoga is also more popular than table tennis, ten-pin bowling, darts, dancing, soccer, cricket, tennis and golf. The proportion of women doing yoga has almost doubled over the period, from 8 per cent to 15 per cent.

The trend is global. According to a *Yoga Journal* report, 20.4 million people practise yoga in the US, up from 15.8 million in 2008. The yoga market is now worth $30 billion in the US and $80 billion globally.

In 2015 yoga was a $1 billion industry in Australia, employing around 12,000 people in 3000 studios. Many studios now resemble upmarket day spas and cost upwards of thirty dollars for a drop-in class. Recently I went to a studio in Sydney's Surry Hills and it was like going to a Gold Class cinema, a masseur and an exercise class all at the same time. Enormous screens ran along the wall, showing stunning scenes shot from helicopters or drones – deer running in the wild, a waterfall cascading into a canyon, a flock of birds fanning out in the sky at dusk – while a guy, not the instructor but her helper, would walk behind us, rubbing our backs and, in shavasana, giving amazing head massages.

Another studio just around the corner was fitted with expensive speakers that vibrated and sent waves of sound through the floor. There was no music, just this vibration that was meant to interact with your breathing and what the teacher termed 'internal currents'. Liberally using the forty-five-dollar bottles of Aesop products under the massive showerhead before drying off with an enormous fluffy towel (it was toasty too, like it had just been taken out of the dryer) and repairing to the tastefully furnished lounge to sip tea or coconut water from the terracotta mini-mug (seventy dollars each), I reflected that yoga – once the practice of some of the poorest people on earth – has moved a long way from its origins.

My first yoga class was in 1999 in a country town – one of those taciturn, cold and tough little settlements that faced the Southern Ocean. Roaring winds rolled in from the Antarctic. It had once been a whaling town, but now operated as a deep-sea port with an aluminium smelter. The town – working class, downbeat, rugged and rough – emitted a sort of spooky vibe. Disquiet, an undercurrent of *something*, was palpable to an outsider like me, alive to nuance and atmosphere in the way only a stranger can be. I had moved to the town for a job, had few friends and no driver's licence. My work was difficult – I was a graduate lawyer, too young and probably too green to do the cases I was given, at once shockingly overworked and underprepared. You should have seen me in court: best debater's voice, ill-fitting suit, my legs – docked unsteadily in too-high heels – trembling until I found my rhythm.

There were long nights working after the office had closed: dictating letters, memos, advices, reading stuff, researching stuff, signing stuff. If it was warm, if it was summer, if we felt like it, a few of us would meet in a car park in the last gasps of twilight and drink or pass around joints. In our cheap suits with our bad haircuts, we'd sit in the gathering gloom murmuring about our files and our cases, complain about our clients and their unpaid fees, but fret about them too. What would become of the shoplifter with the heroin problem? Or the beaten wife too scared to get an intervention order? Or the child in the vicious custody battle? Sometimes we'd go to the local tavern, the Truncheon. It was the sort of place you'd read about in the local paper: a stabbing; intoxicated and unreliable witnesses; dark corners used for drug deals; the service of minors (the large sixteen-year-olds on the football team buying cheap trays of shots).

When I first moved there, I lived in a caravan in a park behind psychiatric services (thin plastic mattress, ill-fitting sheets, the claustrophobic feeling, particularly in summer when the caravan would heat up like a tin can, the scary noises late at night, and the way I would literally wake in fright, and in the morning, the strangeness of putting on a suit, stockings and heels after showering in the communal concrete block). Later I moved to a small house with a garden a short walk from the office. Those Thursday nights doing shots at the Truncheon sometimes ended with my being ill in the caravan park toilets or, once I got a house, in the back garden under a bright spill of stars.

But I was twenty-three and always felt okay the next day. Well, I thought I was okay. But these things can burrow in like termites in wood, insides rotting, and you only see the damage years later when the structure falls apart.

That year, the year I first discovered yoga, I was so lost. I had no idea what I was doing or where I was going. I felt constantly incompetent, out of my depth, socially outside of things, trapped in the town, anxious about the future. (*Was this it, was this what I had been studying so long for?*) That year I put on 15 kilograms, probably from the stress, the drinking, the sedentary work, the despair I saw and felt: the in-and-out of the same cast of characters from court and jail, the unpaid fines, the active warrants, the antipathy of the police, the cynicism of the lawyers, the desolate town and the way the bitter winds would blow down the main street in winter and shut you in for months on end.

In that remote coastal town at the start of the new century, there was no wellness scene; there was no Lululemon, or cold-pressed green juices or $150 yoga mats. The town didn't even have a bookshop. But it did have yoga. The people in that first yoga class I attended seemed down on their luck – ageing hippies with large, soft bodies who moved slowly through the poses and breathed noisily, like Frank Booth from *Blue Velvet*, sucking hard from an oxygen canister. But my fellow country yogis were, in their way, ahead of the zeitgeist. They practised yoga, meditated, grew their own vegetables and pickled them, saw naturopaths, believed in organic – all the things the Bondi crew commodified and paid big bucks for twenty years later, calling it 'wellness'. Nothing is ever new.

In yoga class, everyone wore woollen tracksuits or their gardening clothes. Some of them even wore jumpers. At the end of the class, we covered ourselves in hospital-grade blankets, pulled from a tall cupboard before meditation. The blankets smelt stale and when you unfolded them a cloud of dust would rise, yet being under them was oddly comforting. Nothing about the class was a fashion statement.

The teacher – I still remember him so clearly – had a completely different body shape from all the sporty guys in town. More wiry pipe-cleaner than brick shithouse, he was lean with a straight spine and a small pot belly, like a newly pregnant teen. When he did side angle pose I could see his ribs through his T-shirt. I went with my housemate and we giggled on the way home. *What was that thing he kept saying about 'Ted's arse Ana'? What was with that? Who was Ted? What was his arse like?* We didn't know then about Sanskrit, that he was saying 'Tadasana' (mountain pose) or what any of the poses meant – just that every now and then he'd say 'Ted's Arse Ana' and the class would stand to weary, still attention and settle their laboured breath while we giggled and smirked.

When I was in the studio, the world outside – which seemed stressful, harsh, threatening and hard – would soften and sink. The moon shone in through the high windows; there were candles but no music, just the steady pull and swoosh of the container ships leaving the port and their low, long horns blasting out in a nautical minor key.

Yoga meant moving in a different way from what I was used to. It wasn't the fast, tight spring of running, or the jarring stop/starts of netball, the hard floors, taller girls looming over you with their right arm outstretched in your face like followers at a fascist rally, the taped nails and shrill whistles, the spotlights and cold nights.

This was gentle and strong, challenging and yielding all at once – just you and your body, no balls or whistles. I was moving things I hadn't thought about moving before – the inside of my upper arms and my side waist and the inner thigh and the shoulder muscles. After that first yoga class (or lesson, really; it was my first of thousands of lessons), I experienced a feeling I'd never really known before. It was a deep, sleepy and peaceful yet alert feeling, like I'd woken up in another, less fractious kingdom. People talk about an amplified version of this when they take opioids. The

Berlin Wall you didn't even know you had within you falls. (The divided self heals, and only when that happens do you even know it was divided.) Boundaries collapse. Aches and irritations disappear. My whole body coursed with a new and different energy; an inner tension was relieved and I felt attached or at least connected to my physical self in a way that I never had before. That first night I slept so soundly and deeply, it was like every other night of my life had been serving me an inferior product – a sleep without peace.

The spiritual stuff and the Sanskrit would come later, with other teachers. This first time was all about the body.

Since my early twenties I've been going to yoga – sometimes a lot, sometimes a little. But I've always been going to yoga. I usually carried a tote bag around with me containing soft, loose clothing, in case I passed by a nice-looking yoga studio on the way home from work, and decided to drop in for a drop-in class.

I went to yoga in New York, in London, in Berlin, in Bali, in Texas. I went on yoga retreats to Sri Lanka, Indonesia, Healesville, the Blue Mountains, Hawaii and Thailand. I went to yoga in country towns and in Midtown Manhattan. I did yoga outside and inside, in jungles, deserts, gyms, office conference rooms, bedrooms, basements, bars, church halls and in RSL clubs, on beaches, on the grass, on concrete, floorboards and sand.

I did yoga even when I didn't speak or understand the language spoken by the instructor, when I was sick, and when I was hungover. I did it when I was happy and sad. Fat and thin. Fit and out of shape. Broke and rich. Searching and satisfied.

I wasn't aligned to any particular school. I did Bikram, hot yoga, hatha yoga, kundalini, vinyasa flow, sound yoga, urban yoga, hip-hop yoga, aerial yoga and heavy metal yoga. I had Hindu, Muslim, atheist, African-American, English, French, Italian, Spanish, Australian, American, Indian, Indonesian and Polish teachers. They were young, old, somewhere in between – hundreds of yoga teachers. I did it all. I did it everywhere. All the time. With everyone.

What results did I get after all those hours of yoga? Well, very little, actually. Apart from my intensive time doing Bikram, it never made me particularly lean – although I always felt more supple after. I just never really got good at it. All those hours did not result in any kind of improvement. I've learnt the hard way that I'll never advance to advanced – I'll always be checking the timetable for the yin class, the beginners, the basics, the essentials. It turns out that doing something for 10,000 hours doesn't necessarily make you good at it; it just means you have spent a lot of time on it. For me, yoga was a Sisyphean experience in which I was always struggling to climb the foothills but never really making it to the middle reaches of the range. I was frequently bored, and often frustrated. My body, particularly my arms, hips, shoulders and back (everything above my knees, essentially), lacked the basic flexibility to get into a lot of the poses. I can – still! – barely sit cross-legged. I can't put my hand on the ground in triangle pose. I can't do shoulder stand or headstand (but I can do 'legs up the wall'.) I'm always having to stop and rest, always having to break for water, always making bargains with myself. *If I go into child's pose now then I'll give it a proper blast of energy at the end.* Or: *Maybe if I just do a half push-up instead of a full one, no one will notice that I'm not keeping up with the class, or the only one without a tattoo, or the only one wearing cheap sweatpants and a generic T-shirt* (my favourite was the baggy green T-shirt I wore after working for a Labor MP in 2010, which reads MICHAEL DALEY – LOCAL AND ACTIVE).

In an advanced yoga class in Fremantle, the instructor told me not to come back until I learnt the basics. 'But I've been going to yoga for six years!' I told him.

On retreat in Sri Lanka, the instructor, a man of enormous strength, grunted, strained then dropped me onto the ground when he was demonstrating a pose where he had to lift me into a backbend. People watching winced; it was like seeing an Olympian attempt a deadlift and give himself a collapsed disc with the effort. In Bali I injured myself during yoga – not from the practice itself but from not looking where I was going and walking into an offering. Knocking over a candle and a bowl of oil, I skidded across the floor on the oil slick as rows of yogis looked on, trying not to laugh.

But I kept going back because I knew it was good for me. Even if I didn't seem to be progressing – not even an inch further in my standing bow-pulling pose – when I stopped doing it (and I stopped and started plenty of times), I got as bent-over and stiff as an elderly woman. It was like a little taste of the arthritis I was sure was to come.

So I kept going back and I kept sitting on the mat in the back row, gritting my teeth until it was over and I could get my reward – shavasana, known as the corpse pose, when the body feels as if it is sinking into the floor (through the wood, through the concrete, into the soil), when there are waves of energy that dance across my body, like light moving across water, when a deep feeling of peace and a quiet, stillness in the mind descends and the words of Tibetan lama Nyoshul Khenpo Rinpoche spring to mind:

> Rest in natural great peace
> This exhausted mind,
> Beaten helpless by karma and neurotic thoughts
> Like the relentless fury of the pounding waves
> In the infinite ocean of Samsara.

That was me – *beaten helpless by neurotic thoughts*. Wasn't that all of us?

t is 2016 and yoga is my only form of exercise. I've got into a comfortable groove, doing just enough to stop my body from ossifying but not enough to effect any meaningful physical change. My practice is stagnant at around two classes a week, and I despair that I will never, even after fifteen years, go beyond the beginner classes.

Meanwhile all around me, *they* are multiplying – 'they' being the bourgeois boho yogis popping up like gremlins all over my neighbourhood. They are so much better at yoga than me and I wonder what they have that I don't.

For a start, they look different. Most people I see walking around Bondi have stopped wearing proper clothes. Unless you are around the bus stops in time for the morning commute, people dress almost solely in exercise gear – yoga pants, singlet top and hoodie, thongs in the summer, trainers in winter. The look is casual and sporty – but also relaxed and, I don't know … wealthy. As if they are too rich to care about getting properly dressed.

And they must be rich. They're not chained to *the man*, waiting for the bus at 8am, having to wear some scratchy, uncomfortable suit to work. Instead, these are people who have enough time to do lots of exercise classes and enough money to buy the stretchy pants that often cost upwards of $110. They loiter in the aisles of the organic fruit and vegetable shop, their yoga mats hitting me in the face when they turn around. They zip around the narrow streets by the beach on mopeds or bicycles and, after class, gather around the large communal tables of cafes, sipping ten-dollar juice in mason jars or almond milk chai. And they are lean. Not just skinny, but finely muscled. It's a fit-looking leanness.

I see them – bright and early down at the beach with their dogs and surfboards and boyfriends and babies, or meditating on the concrete bit at South Bondi at dawn, or at Icebergs on a Sunday afternoon drinking chilled white wine and eating oysters – and think to myself, *I'll have what she's having.*

This manifestation of wellness encompasses not just good health and vitality but also spirituality and wisdom. It looks casual and effortless. This is the Good Life incarnate. But how to get there? Where to start?

Then, after yoga class one day, I see a flyer in my studio for a six-week program called the Modern Yogi Project. It promises exactly what I have been longing for! It is the transformation from normal, unenlightened schmuck to glowing, well, bendy, wise yogi.

I sign up immediately, pay a couple of hundred dollars and buy a hefty textbook. For the next six weeks I will be practising yoga six times a week, meditating daily, doing a mini-detox, attending Monday-night classes, journalling and undertaking a batch of 'self-inquiry' questions. I will shake up, examine, replenish and re-energise my mind, body and spirit, and then emerge, butterfly-like, a 'modern yogi'. I will also emerge lean. That is the hope, but

I wouldn't be so superficial as to mention it out loud. It is a deeper transformation that is dangled before us.

So day one, Monday night, and we are all sitting in a circle, on bolsters, covered in blankets, holding copies of *Modern Yoga* – the prescribed textbook allocated by the yoga school, Namaste Dudes. There are thirty-two other people in the room – all but two are women. They look glowing, healthy and fit already. They do not need to be here, surely. Everyone is in activewear, with many wearing the expensive multicoloured yoga pants only sold in sizes ten and down. In the middle of the circle is a bowl of fruit, which could be either healthy snacks or some sort of offering. 'Did you bring an offering?' I ask the girl beside me.

Adam Whiting, our facilitator, asks us why we are here. 'Two words, you've got two words,' he says. Adam wears his longish hair in a man bun, is American and is also, as many yoga instructors are, gorgeous. Already he's told us that he doesn't keep his electronic devices in his bedroom and that for the first two hours of his waking day, from 6am to 8am, he doesn't look at social media. He meditates every day, and at 3.33pm, no matter where he is, he stops what he is doing and gives thanks. He says a little prayer of gratitude and invites others who are with him to do the same.

I have so many questions for him already. What does he use for an alarm? Or does he just wake up naturally? How does he resist the temptation to check his emails once he is in the same room as his devices? What does he do for those two hours without his devices? Why 3.33? I raise my hand and ask him a couple of questions (FYI, he has an alarm clock – the old-fashioned, battery-operated kind) but we have to keep moving because all thirty-three of us have to give our names and then answer the maybe unintentionally really existential question of 'Why are you here?'

Why am I here?

WHY AM I HERE?!

The answers tumble out like truncated Zen koans, like unanswered prayers, like fragments of bathroom mirror affirmations, as we go around the circle.

Settling.

Connection.

Believe.

Freedom.

Letting go.

Surrender.

Love myself.

Some of these are answers I wouldn't expect this group of very good-looking and fit people to give (many of the people taking the challenge are already practising yoga three to four times a week). They are words that hint at a dark sort of hinterland, a well of pain, a private struggle.

Self-love. Self-acceptance. On it goes. There is a quiver in some voices.

Yoga, out of all forms of exercise, promises the most in terms of healing: both inside and out. People go to yoga with broken bodies and broken hearts and give themselves up to the practice and its healing potential in the way that they don't in, say, Zumba or CrossFit or F45.

My two words are 'turn up'. Adam laughs, but it isn't really a joke – I am here to turn up. For a start, anyway, what I want from the project is to attend the project. I want to – need to – turn up. I am forever paying for courses but dropping out when my interest wanes. These programs promise on some level to change my life, or start me on a new path, and I would – like tonight – commence them full of energy and commitment but then flag around the start of the second week, before going back to my unhealthy, bad old ways.

This time, though, *this time* will be different.

※

Yoga originated in India in the seventh century BCE. It encompasses physical and mental exercises, breathing techniques and meditation. In the *Bhagavad-gita*, a 700-verse Hindu scripture in Sanskrit, Krishna defines three branches of yoga: karma yoga (the yoga of action), bhakti yoga (the yoga of devotion) and jnana yoga (the yoga of knowledge). Most in the West are aware only of the first of these, also called hatha yoga. According to writer Suketu Mehta in the *New York Times*, our definition of yoga as a purely physical form is erroneous and limiting: 'Volunteering at a soup kitchen is yoga; raising your voice in praise in a gospel choir is yoga; trying to understand how the galaxies shift and why the poor lack shoes is also yoga.'

Modern yoga, as practised in the West today, is predominantly a physical practice, comprising a series of shapes, poses and breathing exercises. But Western yoga has evolved into a philosophical system that makes suggestions for ways of living and provides a framework for personal growth, reacting to the world and taking responsibility. Due to these doctrinal elements, for many it is less an exercise class and more like religion.

In many ways, yoga is the perfect pastime for our age – the meditative elements give us the opportunity to find peace and stillness in this increasingly hectic and crowded information age, the instructional bits (which I refer to as 'nuggets of truth') give moral lessons in the absence of traditional religion, while the stretchy, bendy, sweaty physical stuff is a great way of countering eight, nine, ten hours a day spent hunched over a computer.

I like yoga teacher and blogger J. Brown's fairly straightforward assessment of why we should do yoga:

> The ultimate goal of yoga is to be well and appreciate life.
> The breathing and moving exercises we do are nothing more
> than a way of easing discomfort and encouraging conducive
> perspective. In turn, practice also tends to facilitate
> intimacy, strengthen relationships and make life more
> enjoyable. This practical application of yoga has always
> existed and ought not be obscured by zealots or profiteers.

Of which – like in every area of the wellness industry – there are many. But more on that later.

On that first, cold Monday night, Adam moves about the semi-darkened room, talking about the next six weeks. It won't be all smooth sailing, he says. Around week three or four 'it's going to be, "Holy shit, I'm tired and I can't focus on meditation," and all these things are going to be coming up and there's going to be a sense of failure. Throw that away right now! We are using the asana to move towards unwavering contentment, bliss and peace.'

The asana he is referring to is the physical aspect of the practice – the poses, such as downward-facing dog.

'We self-understand through yoga. The tools yoga will teach us can create an enlightened life, and an enlightened life means a fulfilled life – to touch into unwavering contentment. It's crazy to think that's possible, to have this unwavering contentment deep inside throughout the unending turbulence of life. We're going to talk about how to access this.'

The access is mainly through yoga and meditation, though Adam stresses that the meditation is the main game, and he'd prefer us to miss a yoga session than stop meditating daily. Meditation, he says, 'is like taking a bullet train to bliss'. Through meditation you can connect with the 'animating force that moves all of us and connects all of us on earth. If you follow your heart and the laws of the Dharma, that (collective) energy is there to do your bidding. When that happens, the path is laid out and the universe unfolds.'

Adam mentions the poet and philosopher Ralph Waldo Emerson and his belief that 'the world makes way for the man who knows where he is going'.

'Sounds amazing, like "yeah, I want that". But what it means is that you have to have a meditation practice, preferably before the sun rises. Wake up at 6am and don't touch any electronic devices until 8am.'

I contemplate buying a digital alarm clock. The first thing I do when I wake up, before my eyes have even properly opened, is check Instagram, then Twitter, then Facebook, then emails. Repeat. The social media cycle of my day is an unhealthy feedback loop of consuming, commenting, then posting content back into the vast, relentless digital matrix. The cycle starts early and finishes late. I usually do one or two Instagram and Facebook posts a day, but on Twitter I am nuts. Since 2009 I have tweeted 45,000 times in a sort of digital and public extension of my internal monologues and half-formed thoughts. I wish I could banish the phone from my bedroom, like Adam has. Right now the little screen is my good morning and my goodnight. I sleep with it beside me. Checking it is an addiction – but, of course, I'm not the only one.

On day two, I start with a yin class. I like yin. It's soft and slow and when it's over, I have usually dropped into a lovely soporific state. Poses are held for forty-five seconds to two minutes, or longer if you're advanced. Heavy-limbed deep sleep and sweet dreams follow. The class involves no sudden moves, no exertion; instead you drape yourself over cushions, folded-up blankets and bolsters like you are an injured ballerina fallen to the floor. The stretch – which the instructor keeps referring to as working the fascia (the connective tissue) – can feel deep and juicy.

I had forgotten how soothing yin could be. An acoustic piano plays from the instructor's iPod while I get into pigeon pose (my head and neck bent over the long bolster, my left knee tucked under me and my right leg stretched out behind me) and I think, *Ah, yes*. I can do this – just lie here, only somewhat uncomfortably, for two minutes on each side, breathing into my slightly rank bolster in the darkened room while the same two chords of a piano circle overhead like some sort of aural string of prayer beads. I am not sweating; I'm not even moving – yet in this almost stationary practice there is still some work happening. My breath is becoming laboured and my glute muscles are starting to ache. This pose is a hip opener. Many teachers, over many years, have said the hips are where you store your emotions and sometimes, in this pose, it's normal to cry. Not just cry but sob. They call it a 'release'.

The room is dark. I listen out for soft sobbing but hear none. I used to not believe the teachers. *What do you mean our hips store emotion?* It sounds dumb, like saying our right leg is the place memories are stored. It's true that the body is a storage facility, but for material things: our fat, blood, bones, organs, cells. Even if you accept the premise that our bodies store emotion (according to author Louise Hay and scientist Bruce Lipton, physical symptoms are evidence of what is going on in your unconscious mind), why the hips?

Wellness website Naturally Savvy calls the hips 'the body's junk drawer'. They are the body's stabilisers, 'but they also serve as storage units that house sad memories, financial fears, relationship woes and family issues. By taking the time each and every day to focus ample attention on the hips, you'll release anxiety, fear, depression and sadness.'

Okay … but what is it about leaning deeply over your calf for two minutes in a room full of strangers that causes these old, stored emotions to be released? It seems witchy, superstitious, pseudo-science.

Yet sometimes, after a very bad week, I've bent my body over my calf – just like everyone else in the class – and felt a spontaneous welling, something not coming from my hips but from my belly, and just started sobbing, naturally, as if a valve has been opened. One pant leg is sopping wet, getting covered in snot and tears. You're down there, your face mashed against your leggings, back and belly quaking, and you can feel the sadness move through you, less like a dance or an exorcism and more like the back-and-forth pull of a king tide breaking on a retaining wall. You hope the aural piano loop or the Bon Iver or Damien Rice song they always play is loud enough to mask the sounds. You hope everyone else in the room is also sobbing so that it drowns out your own noises. In the dark, across those long minutes, where parts of you are simultaneously stretched and compressed, something is being released.

I ask Adam Whiting about the connection between emotion and the physiology of poses such as pigeon. Why do people get teary during this pose?

'I did a little bit of research about why that is, past the surface level of releasing muscle of the hips, which allows for a better loco-motion,' he says.

Adam thinks we can look at the phenomenon in a few different ways. From the perspective of the chakra system, 'if there is a blockage of the root chakra, prana or energy can be released into the body when we stimulate the area with movement, intention, stretch or awareness.' This can result in a release of emotion or sensation. But there is also the physiological release:

> If you look at the musculature of the iliopsoas (which
> gets worked during hip openers), it's amazing how
> dynamic it is. It's been called the muscle of the soul.
> The lower portion comes into contact with the femur,
> which has to do with movement; the mid portion runs
> behind all the reproductive and digestive organs; the
> upper portion attaches into the vertebrae and is deeply
> connected to the diaphragm. This muscle comes into
> play in locomotion, digestion, reproduction, protection,
> breathing and the autonomous nervous system.

It's one of those muscles that can be consciously
connected to the nervous system but can also bypass the
conscious thoughts of the brain and move more towards
the reptile brain. So to be able to manipulate this muscle
in a yoga pose is really important.

Despite being not very good at yoga, over the years I have felt
that it's been beneficial, for the reasons Adam touched on – you
are moving parts of your body that were previously stagnant, and
stimulating blood flow. Yoga has helped me sleep better, and seems
to balance out my equilibrium. I like that it forces me to concentrate for an hour or more, and then at the end, gives me the space
to let go.

I need the discipline. I am always overthinking things, hyper-
stimulated yet unable to focus. I have poor attention to detail and
am prone to alternate bursts of laziness and anxiety. Tests on the
internet indicate I have adult ADHD but I've never sought treatment. What if they gave me Ritalin, like a child who can't focus in
maths? And anyway, haven't I always been chaotic and disorgan-
ised, ever since I was a child? Hasn't my energy always been – as
one Covent Garden tarot-card reader put it tactfully – 'scattered'?

There have been years when I couldn't seem to hold anything
down. Jobs came and went. Men came in and out of my life. Crushes
flush with potential were regularly crushed. I was occasionally
loaded with cash after selling a few articles – mostly celebrity
interviews or long think pieces about youth – but mostly I was
poor and living beyond my means. I had thirty-five superannuation

accounts, each with about ten dollars in them, the principal dwindling each year due to administration fees. Throughout my thirties I lived like an aristocrat fleeing various corrupt regimes and angry creditors, moving from one borrowed manse to the next. *First I'll take Manhattan* ... There were thirty or more houses: Barcelona, London, Berlin, New York, Sydney, Melbourne. I was travelling all the time, but it was haphazard, without a plan. I was a restless romantic, somewhat despairing, but mostly celebrating my ability to be on the move.

I spent ten years – more – flying by the seat of my pants, exhilarated, but also exhausted. My friends could be charmed by my charm, and they liked the crazy stories, but wasn't the hot mess stuff starting to wear a bit thin? I mean, really, how many times could one person lose their wallet? Or leave their laptop sitting on the table in a cafe? Or lock their keys in the house where they'd also left their phone and wallet? Or lose their credit card at a music festival?

It's like I need something, some sort of practice, some sort of rigorous regime, to hold me down and make me, in yoga parlance, more grounded. And if it makes me thinner as well – well, that's a total bonus.

The Modern Yogi Program, with its daily classes, meditation and journalling, is fairly time intensive, like a part-time job. It means going out less or going out at times that work around the yoga schedule. 'Let's meet at 8.20am for breakfast – I'll have finished my essentials class by then,' I tell my friends. Or: 'I can meet at 7.45pm for dinner, somewhere close to the studio.' The yoga timetable becomes the organising principle of my life over the next six weeks. I refresh it constantly on my phone, and carry a hard copy wherever I go. No matter what, I have to go to six classes a week.

Adam says that unless we're feeling unwell or injured, we should try to make the majority of classes vinyasa – the energetic, dynamic power classes where you sweat a lot. The hard yakka. It is also the kind that will give you more of that lean yogi's physique. Yin is a once-a-week treat, a Sunday night wind-down.

By day three I have to force myself to go to vinyasa, even though I don't feel fit, flexible or coordinated enough. I can't cheat and just do six weeks of yin. We have to account for our attendance on a whiteboard at Namaste Dudes. A row of blanks beside my name is both the motivator and the reproach.

Vinyasa is tough. It's a flowing, dynamic form of yoga that links movement to breath. The poses require a mixture of strength, flexibility, agility (to get down low, then bounce up high), concentration, balance, a strong core and cardio capacity. The benefits of vinyasa include increased flexibility, mental focus, cardiovascular conditioning and muscle development. It also burns more calories than the other, slower forms of yoga such as hatha or yin.

I pick a vinyasa class that I hope will be sparsely attended. It's the middle of the day at the Bondi Junction studio. I stay down the back, feeling irritable and tired. My fellow yogis – as usual – look like part-time models and are unsmiling and focused, wrapped in their personal insulation of wellness. I tune in to my body and notice all that I cannot do. My left side is incredibly locked up and stiff. In a cross-legged position the knee of my left side floats up in the air, resisting any downward movement, as if it is being held aloft by a floatation device. Bounce, bounce, bounce. What goes up will not come down. My hips lock up at a certain point, like a rusted compass. I cannot move anything down further. After sixteen years, even after sixteen years, I am about as flexible as a wooden board. It's hard not to feel envy as I watch the woman in front of me transition gracefully, without breaking a sweat, from a standing forward bend to crow pose – a balancing pose where all your body weight is essentially on your wrists and forearms. I leave the class sweaty, spent and still irritated, thinking maybe bodies are a certain way, anatomy fixed, bones fused at certain angles, and all the yoga in the world won't change a thing.

Week one of Modern Yogi passes in a blur of yogi-related activity, each day dictated by the studio timetable, each morning vaguely stressful as I try to squeeze in fifteen minutes of meditation. But after a week, I do begin to notice some physical changes. It's the coldest day of the year, all of six degrees when I wake up. My flat is unheated. But when I get out of bed, I'm bending down and picking things up off the floor with an ease I've not felt before. I've unstiffened, like someone's coated my insides with oil. While I'm not completely lubricated of joint, the difference is noticeable after six days and five classes. Maybe the trick is to slam a heap of classes in a row rather than do years of low-level yoga, attending once or twice a week.

The meditation is also becoming a habit. Adam's passion for it is infectious, and it's nice to do if you are not in a hurry to be anywhere. Sitting up in bed during the bright, short dawns I close my eyes and fifteen minutes later, when I open them, it's morning. I go to the kitchen and put the coffee on.

But if I don't do it first thing in the morning, things unravel. The meditation practice becomes ragged, stressful and uneven. One day, having slept in, I try to meditate on the train. There are people talking on their mobile phones, announcements, and the self-conscious feeling of doing something private in a public space.

Will my meditation end up on Snapchat? I look very holy, like I'm about to receive my First Communion. My hands folded in my lap, eyes closed, lips soft in an almost smile. But I'm conscious too of missing my stop and ending up in Jannali so I keep opening my eyes every time the train pulls to a stop: Edgecliff, Kings Cross, Martin Place, Town Hall. On the train, the practice becomes a micro-meditation, infused with stress.

By the seventh day I return to yin, my limbs feeling light and loose. The yin class is familiar now, like a cave or cupboard where everything is folded in and slowed down. There's the sense of the Sabbath about it – this is the day to rest, to put the phone away, to have a meal with family and friends and end it all with a slow, lovely yoga class.

On Friday in that first week, in a move that shocks just about everyone, the citizens of the UK elect to leave the European Union. The teacher, an Irishman, references Brexit in his 'nugget of truth' sermon about forty-five minutes into the class. We are in pigeon pose, bowing to an unknown deity. I am not crying. 'You might not like change. You may resist change,' he tells us, walking around the heated room. 'You may not agree with it. You may think the change is a bad thing. A very bad thing. But change has happened. It's happened and you can't do anything about it. To resist it is pointless.' His voice is heavy, sorrowful, and he sighs. 'It is what it is.'

As in life.

More than any other activity or form of exercise, yoga has the power to be transformative. You could call the cycling scene or the running scene a *way of life* because people do it obsessively – it's where their friendships, recreation and identity can be found. But yoga incorporates a spiritual dimension that other exercise routines don't have. As Adam said, 'We are using the asana as a way to move towards unwavering contentment, bliss and peace.'

Those, my friend, are big promises.

Sometimes I need convincing about the spiritual stuff. Some teachers impart wisdom and after their classes I feel like I've learnt something important. But other teachers – mainly in the gym chains – fumble with the spiritual aspect of yoga. They don't really know the philosophy from which yoga is derived, or just don't have the language for it. Or maybe they lack the depth. They are doing classes at the gym, subbing for someone when they should be teaching Pump, Zumba or water aerobics. (It reminds me of something the late journalist A.A. Gill wrote of India: 'Plenty of Westerners come to pick through its jumble for something off the peg that fits; they do yoga as exercise, which is a bit like walking the stations of the cross as aerobics.')

After one particularly aerobic vinyasa practice, a teacher with a platinum bob and hot-pink leotard got us to do a visualisation: 'Okay, you're in a lake – I mean, *by* a lake, you're by a lake and you are in a beautiful house. It's a multi-million-dollar house – lots of glass and the sun is streaming in. Feel that sun on your face. Now you're in a car – a Ferrari. It's going really fast and you've got the top down and the music blasting!'

Some things they say are outright lies, ridiculous concepts that seemed to clutch from the air various New Age-y, spiritual things and then try to glue them together with random bits of pseudo-physiology, things that make no anatomical sense. Like: a seated twist pose rinses out your kidneys. Or: this pose massages your liver. Does it? Does it really? Prove it. The best teachers aren't always the most flexible ones – they are the ones who've been soldered through some sort of fire, and have come out the other side with hard, sweet wisdom that demands to be shared.

Adam is a great teacher. He doesn't lay the nuggets of truth on too thick, but when he does impart something it seems to come from an authentic place. One day after class we have lunch at a vegan place in Bondi and he tells me how he came to be a yoga teacher.

It all started in September 2001, when Adam was a teenager and fresh out of music school, where he had studied classical guitar. He got a job working for an insurance agency in downtown New York. The job, his first in the city, wasn't too onerous. It mostly involved entering insurance policies into a computer. The commute, however, was more problematic. Getting the subway in from Queens each day, he had to walk past Ground Zero to get to work. There were loudspeaker announcements being made about explosions going off, there were flyers with missing people dotting the landscape and dust everywhere.

Then, about eight months into the job at the insurance agency, something strange happened. On his way down to the ground floor, Adam freaked out in the elevator.

'The elevator doors opened to the lobby and I took a step out and got the worst vertigo – and I was against the wall,' he recalls. 'A good friend got me on the train to Queens and I got home okay. But the dizziness kept coming back, worse and worse. At first I thought it was something I was eating, dehydration, sinus, or something like that.' Symptoms started piling up: 'Numbness in my legs, headaches, trouble sleeping. I started thinking it was something serious.'

Adam went to a GP and a neurologist and they did the whole gamut of tests – spinal tap, X-rays, MRI, scans. They found nothing. Finally a doctor said, 'Your body is healthy but your spirit isn't.' He was ultimately diagnosed with post-traumatic stress disorder. Doctors in New York were seeing waves of similar symptoms following the events of September 11.

Adam was put on antidepressants and anti-anxiety medication for six months and told to come back at the completion of the course. The meds worked, and while he was happy to be symptom-free, 'the next part of the journey was healing myself without pharmaceuticals', he says, as they had a dulling effect.

Then he found meditation. But it didn't come easily. 'I was so guarded from panic attacks and anxiety that the process of meditation couldn't really find a seat – I couldn't really let go enough. I felt so unsafe in every aspect of my life that when I sat down in stillness, all I ever felt was terror.

'I went to an asana teacher and she said, "You've got to get into the physical practice of yoga first."'

He did and 'it was a really deep physical practice, really heart-based':

> It was in this that I felt the hard shells, the outer layer, start to melt. The physicality of the practice quietened the inner dialogue – but for me it was moving into meditation after asana. I remember the effects of the meditation clearly. It was a ninety-minute yoga class then thirty minutes' meditation afterwards – and the feeling was *you're safe*. The feeling – I hadn't felt it for so long – it was beyond words.

⁂

It's the start of week two when a bad bout of anxiety hits me: a week of short days, dark skies, rain showers thrown across the sky like a veil, my body aching from all the exercise. Before our regular Monday evening Modern Yogi meeting (which is like a mixture of a sharing circle and a university tutorial), I'm in a coffee shop drinking chai, when suddenly I'm gripped by what can only be described as deep dread. Something bad is about to happen, I can feel it. Someone I love is about to die, I can feel it. This isn't paranoia, this is intuition. This intuition feels almost grossly physical – it's all sensation.

I sit in the cafe as if waiting for the anxiety to assume physical form and pull up the chair beside me, have a talk, tell me some really scary things. 'Are you ready?' the dread feeling seems to ask. 'Because you need to be ready. The thing you fear the most is coming.'

The chai getting cold, I sit there for as long as I can, waiting for the stranger to turn up and take his seat. I breathe like we learnt in meditation class until my heart rate slows down. No one takes the seat. I walk to the studio just in time for the discussion group – we are talking about what we are resisting in life that is blocking us from joy.

The theme of the week is 'Choose'. Our booklet says, 'At any time, regardless of the circumstances, you can make the choice to be joyful, so start right now.'

The anxiety and dread are now nestled like a new organ in some cavity in my body. *Don't think you can stay*, I think but do not say.

After class in week two, I count the nights I've been away this year: more than 100 and it's only the start of June. I need to slow down. But, oh, the places I've been and the things I've seen! I've swum with manta rays at midnight in a warm sea off Hawaii, ballooned over the Great Sandy Desert at dawn, ridden a Harley around the base of Uluru as the desert sun came up, climbed the rim of Kings Canyon, which looked to my eyes like the crater of a red moon. I've swum in a wild billabong on an Indigenous cattle station in the west of Cape York, I've seen flocks of rare birds scatter across skies so large that the human field of vision is inadequate for the task, drunk a strange mushroom drink with strangers in a jungle in Thailand and danced in the twilight to Sting! I've wandered the streets of Georgetown in Penang, looking for a mystical cafe where you take a selfie and they put it on your coffee foam.

I've put in a bid on a house I've only seen once for five minutes in a town I was passing through, maybe ending decades of renting and the prolonged adolescence of share houses. The house is old, like 1860s old, with warped glass windows, sloped ceilings, rough unpolished floorboards and vines that run across the verandah. At dusk kangaroos graze out the front, and the only sounds around for miles are the birds, the frogs in the creek and the passing train. I spend hours staring at the pictures on realestate.com.au, willing it to be mine, despite all the obstacles and impracticalities (it's in the country, I don't drive, etc. etc.). I cannot get it out of my head.

Desire is everywhere that winter, bursting from me like a geyser. I've fallen in love after a brief meeting with a guy at a party. My phone is running hot with his text messages and I'm texting back until the pads of my fingers hurt. I'm using all the emojis. My phone is constantly threatening to run out of charge. I can see when he's typing on his phone to mine, the dots appearing like bubbles of someone underwater using up all their air.

The whole thing is exhilarating and exhausting but takes place in some virtual space where we are meeting but not meeting. In the nuggets-of-truth sermons at the end of class, a common theme is to embrace uncertainty. We don't know what the future holds, what the outcome will be. But, man, it is hard.

I go out after a strong yoga class on Tuesday night, where in the shavasàna I'm actually panting and my ponytail is damp with sweat. It's a restaurant opening in Paddington. I meet my friend Tim there and tell him I'm so anxious I can't sleep, that I feel speedy and scared – and that the yoga and meditation, while good, is not making the anxiety go away. 'But at least I have some Valiums from … before. Also, I've put in an offer for a house – somewhere or other!'

He suggests I have a week not drinking, eating lots of fruit and vegetables and getting more sleep. 'But keep up the yoga and meditation.'

'Yeah, yeah, yeah,' I say. We're on the second level of the restaurant, the uneven terraces and hushed backstreets of Paddington spread like a patchwork quilt before us. All is quiet out there. Who says money never sleeps?

Someone comes around with a tray of cocktails – Bellinis, by the look of them. The liquid around the massive ice cubes is an amber light. That first sip is miraculous. The anxiety just dissolves like aspirin in a glass of water. And so I take my medicine.

The next day we sit in that circle in the yoga studio, the fruit in the middle (I have figured out by now that it's for eating – it's not an offering). It's winter. People are in yoga gear with shawls and ponchos around their shoulders.

Adam looks around the circle. 'Meditation – how are people enjoying it?'

His question gets an enthusiastic response – from some.

'My alarm is set for 4.45am each morning,' says one woman in shiny leggings with a pineapple print. She has boot camp at the beach, then a long commute, and now meditation – which she does after boot camp but before work. Unlike me, she does not try to meditate on public transport.

But although many of my classmates are getting up early to meditate, they aren't finding it easy. No one is having difficulty fitting in six seventy-five-minute yoga classes a week, yet when it comes to meditating for fifteen minutes a day, suddenly we 'don't have enough time'. Maybe it's because the results aren't physical – it's not something we or anyone else can *see*.

For Type A personalities – or, really, anyone who has an over-stimulated 21st-century mind – meditation can be frustrating. After all, it looks like a bad use of time. You're not doing *anything*; you're just sitting there. You're not even meant to think things through – like what you're going to cook for dinner.

'My mind won't stop talking,' says one Englishwoman. There are nods of agreement around the circle.

'The chatter is just as important as stillness,' says Adam. 'If you don't have the chatter, you won't be able to recognise the stillness. The calm between the storms of thought.' He tells us about monks who meditate for hours, only to achieve one pure second of silence. The thing is just to accept where you are. 'Chatter happens; right now I'm turbulent. You undulate back and forth. But once you hit that part of meditation where there's stillness, there's nothing like it in the world.'

There are more questions.

'Is being asleep meditating?'

'No.'

'Can you meditate when you are drunk?'

'Sometimes you've got to tick that box.'

'What about exercising before you meditate?'

'If you can burn off the top layers of energy before you meditate, that can be good.'

Everyone is focused on the asanas – that is, the physical aspect of becoming a yogi. We are coming into the studio six days a week and powering through the toughest classes, even people who are sick with winter colds. The home practice is harder. Even the Type A personalities seem resistant to the idea of practising outside the studio. I'm the same. At home I've flung a towel on the ground and done two or three downward dogs, then called it a day.

As with Dr Liu and the fasting clinic, we seem to need a task-master, a public space, an appointment. At home, alone, with no supervising parent, we become lazy and apathetic. We lie around, distracted by our devices.

At this point in the modern yogi journey, Adam asks us to be aware of leaking energy, or 'prana'. 'We have to stop the leaking of prana. Our exercise this week – forgive somebody.'

People groan at this.

'One of my pet peeves is when yoga teachers say, "Let it go." It's not just "let it go" – it's a gradual discharge, like taking an electric charge away from it all.' He pauses. A hush has settled. There's a new atmosphere in the room – thick and heavy. We're all thinking about who to forgive, I'm sure of it. People are involuntarily wincing or have a sad, faraway, wistful look in their eyes. Forgiveness is a bitch, but I believe deep down that it will set you free.

'Can you forgive yourself?' asks Adam. 'That's the most difficult.'

By week three I've found my rhythm with the program and am meditating and going to yoga every day. The studio staff know me now and greet me by name. I have my usual spot down the back in the right-hand corner near the door, and make a thorough job at the end of each class of wiping down my sweat-stained mat – the clean-up and packing away now as much a part of the daily ritual as the rounds of sun salutations. The anxiety is still there, but I move around it. There's a mid-morning vinyasa class with a teacher whose name is Karma, a whole class on shoulders that leaves me aching for days, a class on twisting our 'side waists' after which I feel pleasantly wrung out, cold meditating mornings, being on the phone many times a day to my mortgage broker, who keeps on requesting tax returns and letters from my employer and bank statements, afternoons at the beach when it's too chilly to swim but I sit on the sand with a coffee, texting the dude from the party – back and forth, back and forth – and scrolling through the news. A terror attack at the Orlando Pulse nightclub (forty-nine killed, fifty-three wounded), an ISIS supporter driving a 19-tonne truck through the Bastille Day crowds at Nice, killing eighty-six. Days later, ISIS attackers strike in France again, murdering a Catholic priest in his church.

The Turkey coup attempt, 300 dead, 2100 injured. Erdoğan loyalists arrest more than 6000 people, dismiss another 36,000 from their jobs, and torture and rape hundreds more. In Japan a man with a pathological hatred of disabled people breaks into a care home and stabs nineteen people to death. At home, the Australian election campaign is limping to a close, with disillusioned voters having to choose the least-worst candidate.

Even though we're only halfway through it, there's a fear that 2016 is turning into the *worst year ever*. I wonder how closely my rising anxiety is connected to the increasingly feral news cycle, and if my many, many, many times a day checking and refreshing of news websites and Twitter is bad for my mental health.

Although I can't look away from the news (particularly the increasingly bizarre American election campaign), I'm beginning to make positive changes to my life away from the yoga studio. At the start of week three of the program we are asked to focus our energies on 'getting real' and 'focusing on our dreams'.

The *Modern Yoga* booklet asks us, 'In which areas of your life are you making excuses? Where are you hiding? Is there an aspect of your life where you are ready to come clean?' By uncovering the hidden, more shameful places we become a more authentic version of ourselves. The idea of this week is to step back and compassionately, yet with detachment, observe yourself.

I'm a first-person journalist, I've kept a diary for twenty years, I've been on dozens of retreats – I am no stranger to self-observation. Yet still, like most people, I can be dishonest with myself. Being honest can be painful, and it may lead to an acknowledgement that things need to change. And change is hard. Yoga and meditation can assist in this process, we are told. Part of the yoga practice each day is becoming comfortable with uncomfortable feelings, and sitting there without distraction as they wash over you. These feelings could be the uncomfortable physical sensations of getting into or holding a pose, or uncomfortable emotions that might surface during meditation. This week we are taught that eventually these feelings will pass, as long as we – paradoxically – stay with them.

It is tempting to short-circuit the uncomfortable feelings – by checking your phone, for example – but this is a form of cheating. *Are you making excuses? Where are you hiding?* This week we are told we need to *feel all the feels* and not run away.

I'm starting to notice changes that aren't explicitly a part of the Modern Yogi Program, but they flow from it. For example, if I'm doing yoga six times a week, and working really hard, I'm less inclined to eat junk food. My body craves real food and lots of nutrients. For lunch I swap sausage rolls for salads, and I go to a cold-pressed juice place most days and buy a ten-dollar green juice as a treat after class. Wellness – well, this particular brand of wellness – is proving expensive.

There are also some physical changes as a result of a sudden increase in exercise. Yes, I'm actually becoming leaner! Others notice too and the compliments roll in (but my joy at the compliments shows how much work I have to do on letting go of attachments and ego). My friends and colleagues comment that my hair is shinier, my eyes are brighter, my skin is clearer, my clothes are looser. I'm on the way to becoming more like the yogi women in the Bondi organic shop – healthful and glowing, whacking people in the arm with my yoga mat as I turn around to inspect a peach.

And most gratifying of all for this eternal yoga beginner: in only a few weeks, my physical progress in class is off the charts. I notice certain postures are becoming easier. My hips are opening and I can get my knees down further to the floor when we're cross-legged. I'm becoming stronger and more flexible. My legs and arms are getting leaner, my back is starting to feel properly trunk-like and my previously weak core muscles are switching on. My balance is improving, as is my focus, concentration and stamina. The classes go for sixty or seventy-five minutes and I've gone from wishing it could all be over in fifteen minutes to feeling that I could easily do ninety minutes. Two hours even! I marvel at how adaptable the body is. Some days are harder than others, of course, but some classes I just sail through.

Yet curiously I'm also feeling blanker during yoga, like the classes themselves are a meditation where I don't have to think. I switch off. And the sweetest of all? Those shavasanas at the end, where it's almost as if a chemical calm is flooding across me, cutting through the anxiety momentarily like a detergent through grease. I'm not sure if the sudden anxiety I've been feeling is connected to my dramatic uptake in yoga and meditation or is purely a coincidence. All I know is since starting the Modern Yogi Project I'm having trouble regulating. My energy levels are surging and most nights I can only get around four hours' sleep. Maybe all the exercise is short-circuiting my system or messing with my hormones?

A raft of first-person essays about yoga found on the internet share a familiar narrative: that of yoga saving their life, giving them peace, health, wellbeing, purpose and the gift of spirituality in this secular world. They entered the studio at rock bottom – *they were fat, they were broke, they had been dumped* – and after hopelessly struggling down the back of the class, a transformation was made.

In October 2016, I came across an article on xoJane.com that caught my eye. Headlined: 'I Thought Yoga, Meditation and Instagram Could Save Me from PTSD After I Was Raped', the piece was written by Sydney woman Phoebe Loomes. It provided a counterintuitive narrative about yoga, one you don't often hear. She had spent the day ticking all the wellness boxes: up since 6am, a dawn swim, asanas on the wooden deck of the place she was staying at on New York's Rockaway Peninsula. She recalls giving very yogic advice to someone that day: 'You can overcome anything. Everything you need is inside you.'

That night Phoebe was drugged and raped by a bar manager. Initially, after the attack, she returned to her routine of daily yoga: 'I was angry about what had happened to me, but I was determined to continue on my path to enlightenment … So I committed to stop myself from thinking about it. I repeated my mantra – let go – whenever I caught myself thinking about what had happened to me.'

I contact Phoebe and arrange to meet her for lunch in Sydney to hear more about what role yoga played in both helping and harming her.

She tells me why she got into yoga in the first place. 'Aged twenty-three I went through a really bad break-up. I used alcohol and drugs to cope and it wasn't working for me. I wanted to start exercising. I was much heavier, so when I started doing yoga

I lost a lot of weight really quickly – 16 kilograms over the course of about eighteen months.'

It wasn't purely from exercise, Phoebe says. The place where she was doing yoga encouraged veganism, so she adopted that as well. She didn't find the change in diet hard because, just as I have found, 'when you are exercising and feeling healthier and seeing results it becomes easier to restrict your diet':

> Looking back, I had major issues with eating and control. I couldn't control much else in my life. I lost my social life with that break-up, and being able to spend my evenings at a yoga studio was liberating because I didn't have to think about what else to do. I found this new community. I was a bit nuts and looking back I was a bit orthorexic but it wasn't just food – it was spirituality as well. I found a lot of answers. It wasn't a bad thing.

Then, America, and that night. Phoebe was back on the mat three days after she was raped. For a few days she felt traumatised, but then worked herself up to get over it. 'This is the magic of yoga,' she told herself, 'anything can happen to me and I will be okay. I have the whole toolkit, I can cope.'

The impact of the rape didn't start to hit until five months later, when Phoebe was back in Australia and attending a yoga retreat.

'Everyone I did yoga with had trauma and anxiety and I was listening to their stories and I was thinking, "You don't know what trauma is – you haven't been through anything I've been through."' She felt angry at all of them for taking up her time. Losing your compassion for other people is a common PTSD symptom. 'That's the first time I realised I wasn't coping,' she admits. But Phoebe still refused to properly acknowledge it.

After the retreat her life started to fall apart. 'I started fucking everything up. I lost a lot of friendships because of my anger and inability to be compassionate to anyone. That was hard because such a big part of my yoga practice is to be compassionate, kind and softly spoken and I couldn't do it.'

In the end, a non-yogi friend who'd always been sceptical of her endless positivity called her out on it. 'I was at a friend's birthday at a pub and staring into the middle distance and she was like, "What is wrong with you?"'

Phoebe told her she had been feeling suicidal and wasn't coping.

'It was just very hard for me to accept that I'd been victimised – I had this whole narrative in my life, on Instagram, of being a yogi, and I just didn't want to let it go. It was an identity – and an ego thing.' Phoebe moved in with her friend and started doing intensive psychotherapy for PTSD. That was around two years ago. She still does yoga but recognises its limitations.

'People need that spiritual instruction in their lives. I needed that in my life. I was so lost and I'm so glad that I found the answer – and something divine.' But she acknowledges that expecting yoga to solve all her problems is wrong-headed. 'If I was a Christian and I was raped, I wouldn't look to the church. The problem wasn't yoga – it had solved all the other problems like a bad break-up, but what I went through was so much more serious, and yoga alone can't help PTSD.'

✲✲

All the studies point to yoga as being an excellent tool to help reduce garden-variety anxiety. The Harvard Mental Health newsletter quotes a small German study published in 2005, in which twenty-four women who described themselves as 'emotionally distressed' took two ninety-minute yoga classes a week for three months. Women in a control group maintained their normal activities and were asked not to begin an exercise or stress-reduction program during the study period. Though not formally diagnosed with depression, all participants had experienced emotional distress for at least half of the previous ninety days. At the end of three months, women in the yoga group reported improvements in perceived stress, depression, anxiety, energy, fatigue and wellbeing. Depression scores improved by 50 per cent, anxiety scores by 30 per cent, and overall wellbeing scores by 65 per cent. Initial complaints of headaches, back pain and poor sleep quality also resolved much more often in the yoga group than in the control group, according to the study.

If it weren't for the anxiety, and if I had time and money, this routine of yoga and meditation every day would be the path to vigour, vitality and wellness that I'm seeking. When I did yoga only a couple of times a week, it wouldn't take long – a day, maybe – before I felt 'locked up', fatigued and stiff. In that state it felt as if things weren't flowing – blood, oxygen, my body, my life. Inside and out, I became ... stuck. The Chinese call this chi, but whatever it is, if I didn't exercise every day, I would feel stagnant. Doing yoga every day, I feel the opposite of stagnant – I'm vital. Maybe too vital! And with all this surplus energy I'm going out all the time.

Week three of Modern Yogi Project and there is the Frida Kahlo exhibition opening night at the Art Gallery of New South

Wales, with free champagne and mini burritos and women walking around the gallery in long skirts and their hair piled high on their heads, and later dinner with the Mexican ambassador and a coterie of Kahlo scholars – trays of tequila and bottles of wine, and later, outside, sheets of rain, the streets a hazard, Toto's 'Africa' playing really loud in the Uber on the way to another party in Glebe where everyone is talking about Nauru and the upcoming boring election, the Uber driver saying that he can no longer afford to live in this city but he doesn't know where else to go, and all the while I'm clutching the Namaste Dudes timetable and rearranging my class schedule in my mind (*well, I'm obviously not going to make the 8am class if it's now 3am …*).

Then, midweek in the city, at a methamphetamine forum, drinking too much red wine and eating all the cheese and wondering why anybody would take such a fucked-up drug, without acknowledging my own excessive inclinations. A *Guardian* party in Surry Hills farewelling a colleague moving to India, buying rounds of bottles of wine, trading cigarettes in the courtyard, smoking with our jackets done up high against the cold, and the block of anxiety melting with the addition of each unit of alcohol. All the while my body aches in the best possible way from all the daily movement and stretching, and the bag with the always slightly damp yoga clothes comes with me everywhere. It feels like I'm carrying a bag of wet soil.

The week rolls on. More fun! More parties! More yoga! Blurry Uber rides home, not enough to eat, trouble sleeping, the 4am Valium to bring it all down so I don't have to see the sun come up again. More yoga. More meditation. In some classes I'm dripping so much sweat that I can't see out my eyes. Sweat pours out of my head and covers my hair, which becomes dirty and matted. At home I'm endlessly washing yoga clothes, scribbling in my journal and listening to a lot of Father John Misty and Courtney Barnett, hearing in the lyrics mainly gentle and weary disgust with the world and our objects of idolatry.

By Sunday at 5pm I cannot get out of bed. I'm too tired to move. The rain lashes the windows. The sea is a grey line with white caps in the distance – forming and dissolving, dissolving and forming. The federal election was the day before, and I'd visited all four corners of the city writing about the mood of the people before going to Malcolm Turnbull's terrible victory party at the Sofitel. There was the weird corporate art in the lobby, the three layers of security checks, the bitter champagne and greasy canapés, big televisions covering the count but nobody watching. It gets past midnight. Malcolm takes ages to claim victory – if indeed victory can be claimed – and when he does he's angry and gives a bad speech. The press are all sloppy drunk and getting bored. I get drunk as well, and spend half the night in an upstairs suite with a colleague, talking about the meaning of life and drinking room-service red wine. The rest of the time I'm riding the elevators in between floors, skulking about and staking out secret Tory parties. Girls with taffeta gowns, super-straightened hair and private-school accents are weeping under lobby palms. The boys look sweaty and shop-soiled, anxious and angry – all at once. Somehow, somewhere in the night I lose my credit card. I get home at 2am and wake at 5am to file my story. I consult the timetable, and circle a yin class. No matter what else is happening, I cannot miss yoga. I need to practise six times a week or … or … or … I can't tick my name off on the Namaste Dudes board, I can't morph into this thing I'm destined to be: a modern yogi. A modern yogi with a demanding social life.

Yin is the only option when you're struggling to get out of bed. You can turn up on little or no energy and it will be okay. That night the Irish instructor talks about sides – sides of the body, sides of life. You can't just work on one side – the juicy, loose, flexible side. Does this mean we shouldn't always play to our strengths, but explore our weaknesses with equal vigour? I wonder if it has something to do with the teachings on Monday night, and the self-reflection: 'Are you making excuses? Where are you hiding?' The instructor tells us that in the practice you have to spend time on both sides, that they'll both feel different and be different. Left and right, yin and yang, good and evil, activity and rest. We need to be equally aware of each half and not favour one over the other.

This kind of yoga talk is full of parables and hidden meaning and as you're lying there, open to receiving, you bring to it whatever is going on in your life. It makes me think about my two duelling sides – wellness and hedonism. The more yoga I did, the stronger the hedonic urge. The more meditation I did, the more medication I was taking to help me sleep. It doesn't make sense – unless these are two parts that cannot coexist or unite. My wild side is giving me guilt, which maybe is the most modern trait of all when it comes to being a modern yogi – we'll rise at dawn and drink the organic green juice, but then stay out too late at night drinking cocktails. I'm not the only one. At the studios around Bondi, particularly on a Sunday night, I hear people talking about their weekends – all the coke they had, the nights of two hours' sleep. The yoga class is a corrector to the cocaine. It is the Bondi wellness paradox and I see it over and over again. It's former Olympic swimmer Geoff Huegill announcing that, after serving a six-month good behaviour bond for cocaine possession, he and his publicist wife are starting a health and wellness business.

It's getting hauled out of your house by police during a massive Bondi drug bust while looking pristine in your activewear.

And it's Lisa Stockbridge, an eastern-suburbs blogger and convicted cocaine trafficker, complaining at a hearing about the conditions in prison. According to the *Daily Telegraph*, 'the self-styled lifestyle blogger also said prison food made her hair fall out, gave her migraines and mood swings, all brought on by her many dietary intolerances'.

'I have issues with sugar, wheat, dairy, yeast, anything that is processed,' Stockbridge told the *Tele*.

Bondi sells Australia wellness, with products such as organic soaps apparently borrowing some of the suburb's magic. It also sells Sydney its nightlife. We laugh, but the Bondi paradox is not necessarily hypocritical. Other societies managed to integrate both discipline and excess without seeming schizophrenic or contradictory. Look at the Greeks. Letting loose before knuckling back down has been a way of life since the days of the Greek god Dionysus. There are the Easter celebrations after Lent, there's Carnival and Mardi Gras.

In her 2006 book *Dancing in the Streets*, the writer Barbara Ehrenreich uses the term 'collective joy' to describe group events that involve theatrics, music, dancing and a sense of loss of self. She argues that for at least 10,000 years humans have made space in their lives – at arranged times – for festivals. In Australian Indigenous culture, you see it in rock art – it's there in the ceremonies. For other countries, it's the town square and the maypole, or going into the desert and taking ayahuasca and forgetting your cares for a few days. It's Burning Man and Glastonbury.

'To join in dances, to laugh with the flute, and to bring an end to cares, whenever the delight of the grape comes at the feasts of the gods' – this is the bacchanalian way, Euripides wrote. In losing control, followers lost their self-consciousness and cares in brief, intense frenzies before returning to their highly ordered lives.

These community-based festivals continued right through the Middle Ages and beyond, and invigorated and strengthened communities. Ehrenreich charts how the practice went out of fashion by the 17th century, as puritanism and capitalism smothered our habits of collective joy. Worship became less loud and Pentecostal, and more stifled and silent.

We need to lose the self from time to time – otherwise we'd be driven mad. Once we would try to lose ourselves in love, war, religion or drugs but now we attempt to lose ourselves in the struggle for body, mind and spiritual perfection. We desire to be clean, lean and serene. What is this struggle but trying to overcome death and disease? What is *wellness* but the futile struggle against inevitable loss?

While each morning I am waking at 4am, unable to sleep, I am also checking in with a therapist. She wants to keep an eye on me, worried that while I am becoming a full-on yogi I am also becoming a train wreck. There is the string of crazy nights, a spontaneous decision to buy an 1860s cottage thousands of kilometres from my current home – in a town where I know no one – a lost wallet and cards, the confusion about the dude who keeps texting but is proving elusive in real life, tearing through the Valiums at night, the crying jags, the parties, the cigarettes and the anxiety.

She tells me, 'Meditation and exercise can bring feelings to the fore. The things you need to feel well – meditation, good diet, yoga – are bringing things up, like a sore, coming to the surface.' It's like the detox all over again. I am having a mental healing crisis.

'You should observe the extremes,' she says. 'How do they live side by side? One – wellness – doesn't necessarily cancel the other – hedonism – out.'

'Uh-huh, uh-huh, uh-huh,' I mutter as I take notes in her consulting room, the yoga bag there at my feet, where it always is.

It's now a month into the Modern Yogi Project, and I've banned myself from going out so much. It's raining outside and all week the news has been of the ascendancy of Trump, unarmed black men being shot in America, police being shot by protesters, and a week or more of uncertainty over the election result at home. One Nation leader Pauline Hanson is returned to the Senate on a wave of right-wing nationalist sentiment.

The American yoga instructor leading tonight's class has an accent like Lena Dunham's. The lights are down and the heaters are blasting. I've strained my lower back in one of the poses; I can feel a weak pulsation and am lying on the ground, trying to breathe into the pain, to feel it properly so that I can also feel it pass. The instructor walks around us, talking. 'I've been feeling really down lately,' she says. 'It's mid-winter, it's cold. I'm thinking about all the shitty things that are happening in the world and I've decided there's not enough love.' She reaches down to correct someone's posture. 'People are so sterile. They're afraid to touch each other on the bus. We're all made of the same thing. We're all just cells dancing. Love each other. Be warm. Be kind. If someone is unkind it's because bad things are going on with them. So love them. Show them kindness.'

And even though I am not in a hip-opening pose, and I do not like to touch people on the bus, lying on the studio floor, I find myself crying.

S trong practices are getting easier every time I get on the mat now. I meditate daily, craving it – the mental space, the quiet twenty minutes (we've moved up five minutes from fifteen), the way towards the end everything just empties out and time loses all its tension.

My diet is changing without much input from anyone. There's no program being shoved down my throat, no dietary plan, yet without it feeling like a hardship – without the need for ceremony, ritual, one last binge, the anticipation of future regret – I am letting my old favourite foods go and gravitating towards healthy options. If only I had known it could be so easy.

Things I clung to in the past, my 'favourite' things – dirty burgers, chips, chocolate, pasta, three lattes a day – I just don't feel like any more. One morning I learn the hard way about not eating a massive, cooked breakfast fifteen minutes before class. In the room heated to 30 degrees I can feel the food move up (all that avocado, all that toast and coffee) and the sweat pouring off me is not the cleansing kind but feels toxic, meaty and dense. The worst poses are the inversions and crunches. I spend most of the class lying down, struggling not to throw up.

There is a nutrition aspect to the Modern Yogi Project – a

juice cleanse halfway through, which I don't do. They don't really push it. In the Monday night meeting Adam says he has met yogis who are frequently on juice cleanses, and if you're not careful with the intention behind your cleanse, it can be just another form of eating disorder. I've been down that road before and I'm done with detoxes.

By week five my body is showing signs of wear and tear from all the exercise. Some ancient exhaustion reappears. My left hip aches. I see a physio and he presses his body weight right onto me. I sweat with pain. I have an injury on the left side that he believes is caused by turning off my glutes and overusing my front hip muscles. It's a yoga injury – repetitive rather than sudden, probably from too many warrior poses. When I walk, I feel like an invisible hand is pulling my left leg out of my hip joint (Oh, what a feeling! What a terrible, weird feeling!) but also I'm quite pleased. This means I've joined some elite world – an athlete's world, where people have *sporting injuries*.

I tell people even when they don't ask: 'You may have noticed I'm walking a bit funny ... well, would you believe I'm doing so much yoga that I have *an injury*? Not serious, but still ... I guess that's what happens when you exercise – you know, vinyasa, every day.'

I'm not the only one. A week later I'm getting a pedicure at a nail bar in Bondi (one of the problems with yoga is you spend a lot of time staring at your feet) and another customer recognises me. We chat through the partition of the waxing room. She was also doing the Modern Yogi Project but had to drop out because she hurt her hip.

In the Monday meeting a woman approaches me. I was sharing news of my special yoga injury with the group ('When I walk I hear *click click*'). She is practising every day – 'I'm practically an addict!' – and her hips are gone, both of them. She can't run without feeling like her legs are about to fall off. Some of the women in the course say that if something gets between them and their daily practice they become agitated and unsettled. Injuries don't stop them.

I wonder if it's possible to become addicted to yoga. Surely when different parts of your body 'go', practising through the pain is the equivalent of trying to shoot up into a collapsed vein.

The *New York Times* published a story in 2012 on yoga injuries, interviewing Glenn Black, a yoga teacher of nearly four decades. Black has come to believe that 'the vast majority of people' should give up yoga completely. 'It's simply too likely to cause harm,' he says.

People injure themselves because they have 'underlying physical weaknesses or problems that make serious injury all but inevitable'. Instead of doing yoga they should be doing exercises designed specifically for them, to strengthen weak parts of the body:

> Yoga is for people in good physical condition. Or it can
> be used therapeutically. It's controversial to say, but it
> really shouldn't be used for a general class ... To come
> to New York and do a class with people who have many
> problems and say, 'O.K., we're going to do this sequence
> of poses today' – it just doesn't work.

For a start, he says, most people who are doing one or two classes a week do not have bodies adapted to the poses invented by Indians who squat or sit cross-legged a lot. Instead we are more likely to spend at least eight hours a day sitting behind a desk or in front of a computer. When we then go to a crowded class with people of differing abilities and attempt to twist or land into a position our bodies are not used to, we are vulnerable to injury.

Black says he has seen some 'pretty gruesome hips'. One of the biggest teachers in America had no movement in her hip joints: 'The sockets had become so degenerated that she had to have hip replacements,' he tells the *Times*. Other teachers had such bad backs, they had to teach lying down.

Other injuries detailed in the article include strokes, whiplash-style injuries from moving the head and neck too quickly, cervical-disc injuries, muscle strain, rotar-cuff tears and, in Bikram, injuries related to over-stretching in the heat, including muscle, cartilage and ligament damage.

The sky is the colour of soot – the branches bare and tapping on the window. The lorikeets are still there, bright against the grey. They scream for a bit then fly away. I am waking around 4am most days; I lie there then meditate. At 5am the traffic starts up again – the swoosh of cars, the faraway headlights, the 389 bus turning carefully on the wet road.

My life revolves around my yoga schedule. If I don't practise every day, I feel weird – anguished, even. I get sick with a cold but try to practise anyway, taking some super-strong drugs a friend brought back from the US. They are quite speedy and I don't sleep properly for three nights, but that's okay – as long as I have enough energy to go to yoga.

I get another massage and the pain is almost more than I can bear. The masseur is walking on my back, his hands, rough and strong, are digging into my groin, stretching out my thighs. My body tenses, drenched in sweat. I long for something to bite down on.

On a trip to Canberra I fret – what if I can't find a good yoga studio? In Manuka, I find a studio but it's slow and boring – all middle-aged public servants, by the looks of it – and they don't play the right music. I miss Namaste Dudes and the cool kids there – their beauty and their tight bodies, their fierce dedication and their expensive activewear, the way they greet each other with over-the-top hugs and the way they just seem to live it. I'm not one of them but they give me a living, breathing ideal to aspire to. Some of them have their own Instagram pages, and the Likes gather around their feet like small offerings to a Hindu deity.

But in darker moments I question these wellness idols and ideals that so many of us have chosen to worship. Aren't the modern yogis just flaunting a fairly unrealistic, ath-lean body shape? After all, who has time to go to a ninety-minute yoga class every day? Aren't they just setting the rest of us mortals up for disappointment? Are we just wasting our time and a fair amount of money chasing this elusive thing called wellness? Are we looking in the right places? More importantly – will wellness make us happy?

Even now that I'm doing yoga every day, and regular meditation, I'm finding that it's not making me happier, even if it is making me fitter. There's a definite endorphin high after each class, and the yin classes are calming. But I still feel generally unsettled and anxious – and not grounded at all.

In week six, walking along Campbell Parade on a sunny winter's day after class, I feel tremulous, on the edge of tears, shimmering with barely suppressed feeling. It's 23 degrees in July and everything is too bright and hot. The air is dry and unmoving. The beginner surfers are trying to ride waves that don't have the energy to form. It's a Tuesday and most people are at work. What am I doing with my life? Why am I even here, with only yoga to fill my days? The house purchase is becoming something of a mirage. My mortgage broker can't find a bank that will lend me money. My financial past – earning $100,000 one year and $20,000 the next – confuses them. Outside all is flat and still and hot and golden. I am coming down from my wellness high – from every high. The cottage in the country wasn't the only mirage ... The dude has stopped texting me back. I saw him on Facebook with some other girl, and it felt like being punched. I closed the computer, went into my room and retrieved an old, stale cigarette, which I smoked by the window and cried. I put all that energy into him, only to be ghosted. Romantic rejection doesn't get any easier to bear, even when experienced in the middle of a wellness kick, even when you're looking good.

Walking up the rise from Campbell Parade, I order the nineteen-dollar organic mushroom dish (the 'woodland bowl') from Bondi's uber-cool Porch and Parlour and a ten-dollar green juice. I can Instagram my meal, my juice, and the beach in one #cleaneating #bondi frame. I'm starting to get yoga muscles yet am the saddest-looking wellness person in the wellness cafe.

I've seen other people like me in cafes from time to time, radiating something – something raw and sad and powerful. They sit on a stool at the window or at the edge of the communal table, and the force field, the power of their sadness, creates its own climatic system. I've seen the wellness boys and girls when they thought no one was looking – in the cafe, by the locker, after class, their eyes briefly meeting my eyes in the change room at the studio – and there is sadness there too.

I've seen the same people on Instagram, hashtagged to the hilt with styled bed hair – and I've thought, *How is it possible to be that full of shit? Doesn't it defeat the purpose of all this* work? *For fuck's sake, just be real.*

Meanwhile, the year marches on, and the world outside this beachside bubble is getting madder and meaner. Loads of good celebrities have died way before their time, and there is a sense of standing on the plates of history as they are shifting. The US presidential campaign is in full swing and Republican candidate Donald J. Trump is promising to deport Muslims from the US. He calls Mexican immigrants rapists and criminals and threatens to build a great big border wall. His rallies are electrifying, terrifying, unpredictable and violent. People not prone to hyperbole compare Trump with Hitler. In the UK, the public is fed lies and misinformation by politicians who lack all conviction, and are asked to vote on exiting the EU, the thing set up not just to facilitate movement of people and trade, but also to ensure events like World War I and II wouldn't happen again. Nationalism and xenophobia are on the rise in the West. The war in Syria has caused a refugee crisis of massive proportions. By mid-year more than 3000 Syrian refugees have drowned in treacherous journeys across the Mediterranean Sea. It had been the longest, hottest summer on record. It is now winter, as if autumn had forgotten to arrive. The online world where I spend much of my time is becoming an increasingly brutal space – particularly if you're a woman. I have stopped reading the comments published under my columns for the *Guardian*. The bad ones make me heartsick and I want to keep writing with the exhilaration and freedom that hooked me into the game in the first place.

The market is without morality. Careless market forces will gobble up and transform anything where there might be a profit. For all its hippy, non-materialist vibes, yoga is no exception. An individual yoga studio and its teachers are often only trying to do their best to create a community out of dust – and while it might be a 'caring' community, it is still hooked onto a capitalist system that is making a tonne of money from the wellness industrial complex. People are packed into classes, which are north of twenty dollars a pop; yoga teacher training costs thousands (courses start at around $3000 and can go up to $10,000) and retreats are pricey.

It's not just the studios. Take a look at the market for yoga mats, for instance: according to market research company Technavio, the North American yoga and exercise mat business is expected to climb from a current US$11 billion to US$14.03 billion in 2020 (this is just for the *mat*). Sales of athleisure clothing, including yoga pants, generated US$35 billion in 2015 – an all-time high – making up 17 per cent of the entire American clothing market, according to market research firm NPD Group. The trend is also booming in Australia; research conducted by Victoria University for the Australian Sporting Goods Association predicted that sales of activewear in Australia are expected to continue to grow by more than 20 per cent by 2020.

Yoga pants by Lorna Jane cost $110, and Lululemon's pants are a cult obsession among 'a certain set of gym-minded women and busy moms across the country', according to *GQ* magazine. Lululemon yoga gear is collectable: certain lines of sweatpants or shorts are highly prized, like jewellery or designer dresses.

You can also buy Lululemon prayer beads for $108.

The company has come under fire for prescribing a rigid aesthetic for the people who work for them (young yoga hotties) as well as their customers (at the time of writing, their clothes did not come in larger sizes. They have since expanded their selection). Critics say it defines 'wellness' within a particular aesthetic paradigm.

In an article for Jezebel in 2015, a former (anonymous) Lululemon employee said: 'They co-opt something from yoga and warp it until it loses its true meaning … They mean to be relevant, and instead they manipulate good ideas until they become totally corrupt.'

Churches used to be important. It's hard to understate just how central they were a mere generation ago, particularly if, like my people, you lived in a country town. They were where you made friends, socialised, met your partner, networked for jobs and got assistance when times were tough. If you were poor you could get food, clothes and money; young couples went there for marriage counselling; refugees came for English language lessons. You were born into a church, educated by it and you were buried in it. You kept the cycle going by bringing your children into the church through the sacrament of baptism, and the habit of weekly mass.

Christianity's decline is so sharp as to have fallen off a cliff – in Australia anyway. But just because religion has almost disappeared, it doesn't mean we don't need it. Regardless of whether or not you believe there is a God, organised religion can provide a sense of meaning, ritual and community. We've picked up some threads from old religions but the fabric is now pretty threadbare. So we go off searching. We might try a few different sorts of yoga at a few different studios and see which one suits us, where there might be a good community (it's no coincidence that yoga studios explicitly talk about community when advertising classes). We go to India and find gurus to study under. Like modern monks – but with wi-fi and wheelie suitcases – we go on retreat where we meditate, eat simply, go to bed early and reflect on where we are and where we have to go. Yoga is part of this 'religion-lite' offering.

It's not all bad. The nuggets of truth in many of the Namaste Dudes yoga classes were vital in steering me through this troubling winter. They provided a counterbalance to the grim politics of the year, the disappointments in love, the stress of trying to buy a house – as well as being a way of imparting wisdom, information and a value system that resembled an old-timey church sermon.

We've thrown out most of the old-timey church stuff – yet in its place is a yearning for something bigger and more powerful than ourselves. In the last few years, the public appetite for guidance from the amorphous beast known as the wellness industry has become almost like a mania. I don't think it's too big a call to say that for many young people (mostly young women) yoga and meditation have replaced church as their main form of spiritual sustenance.

For the children of secular baby boomers, born into nothing – no religious tradition, no rituals, no catechism, no theology, no sacred texts – yoga fills a gap. You pay your twenty dollars and you submit to a form of spiritual teaching. What else have we got? Our society is so impoverished that all it can dish up to satisfy our hunger is entertainment and distraction. We gorge ourselves on it. It's not so much satisfying as numbing – and profoundly fucking sad. It's no surprise that a yoga class is the best the mainstream can offer on the spiritual front.

The yogic way of life (physical practice, meditation, self-knowledge, a philosophy, spiritual practice) is definitely not a cult, and definitely not a religion, yet, like fasting, it can have the rigour and the discipline of religious devotion. Yogis in training have to submit to this way of life. To get there fully you have to change not just your body and what you put in it, but also your habits, how you structure each day, your social life, your mentality, thought patterns, your inner life, your intellect, your spiritual beliefs, your friends, your worldview. In other words, you have to change your world.

Instagram has thrown up a whole generation of patron saints who demonstrate how it is done. You follow them. 'Fall in love with taking care of yourself. Mind. Body. Spirit,' they write over a picture of themselves doing crow pose on the sand at sunrise, as the sky flames and water laps. You don't desire the person in the photo. That's not the aim any more. The desire, more carnivorous and impossible, is to *be* them.

The result of all this work on yourself is a feeling that might be described as vitality or some sense of optimum health, fitness, calmness and strength. Your body is humming along tickety-boo, but so are your spirit and your mind. After all, *yoga* in Sanskrit means 'to yoke; join together, pull along'.

But does yoga *yoke us together* in a broader, collective sense? American writer Judith Warner notes a disturbing social trend. Just as the women of the mid-1970s took flight into consciousness-raising groups, the work force, divorce and casual sex, their daughters are also taking flight, but that flight is inwards. 'They're fleeing to yoga,' she writes in the *New York Times*, 'imitating flight in the downward-gazing contortion called the crow position. They're striving, through exquisite new adventures in internal fine-tuning, to feel more deeply, live more meaningfully, better inhabit each and every moment of each and every day.'

Warner glumly concludes, 'There's no sense that personal liberation is to be found by taking a more active role in the public world.' In fact, 'such interiority seems to be a way to manage an unbearable sort of existential anxiety: a way to narrow the scope of life's challenges and demands ... to the more manageable range of the in-and-out of your own breath'.

As a result of this dereliction of public duty, the world then turns a certain way, and not another. What was the election of Donald J. Trump except a manifestation of this abdication of a sort of collective ideal?

In the wellness industry we can self-actualise: follow our bliss and find individual contentment, be the best version of ourselves we can be. The collective has collapsed in favour of the individual. We can't do anything about inequality or the ruined environment or the heating planet – but we can get really, really good at these poses and master all the potential shapes that our body can make. Before Trump we had long stopped marching, and taking our *issues* to the streets; instead we took them to our mats.

Carl Cederström and André Spicer, authors of *The Wellness Syndrome*, argue that obsessive ritualisation of self-care comes at the expense of collective engagement, collapsing every social problem into a personal quest for the good life. Writing in the *Baffler*, British commentator Laurie Penny agrees:

> The slow collapse of the social contract is the backdrop
> for a modern mania for clean eating, healthy living,
> personal productivity, and 'radical self-love' – the
> insistence that, in spite of all evidence to the contrary,
> we can achieve a meaningful existence by maintaining

a positive outlook, following our bliss, and doing a few
hamstring stretches as the planet burns.

In yoga, when we talk about structural problems it is our bodies that we are referring to – the way having short arms might make triangle pose difficult, for example. As for the other structural problems – the patriarchy, income and housing inequality, Indigenous recognition and a profit motive that is destroying the environment – we prefer to look away.

Social change and self-care do not have to be mutually exclusive but I wonder if a greater engagement with the collective could come at a studio level. A good yoga instructor won't necessarily be a political teacher, but the values of love, compassion, kindness, inclusivity and respect that yoga instructors talk about – these are becoming political values in the age of Donald Trump.

Yoga means 'to yoke'. We need to yoke these values found in the studio to politics and public conversation. That's where we start.

But what about the practice itself? Will doing yoga change your life? Or at least give you a lean body? Well, yes. It can.

It's easy when most of our work is so sedentary to become disassociated from our bodies. It's easy to let the disassociation become the dominant way of being. It's there in how we unwind after work – television, boxset binges, large glasses of wine, a beer or tumbler of Scotch, a joint before bed, a trashy novel, hours spent scrolling Facebook or Twitter, getting lost down the internet click hole, all the entertainment, all the numbing, all the distractions. These distractions are the way we push away darkness, sadness, doubt, a nagging sense of meaninglessness or pain. But they also mean that we are not really in our bodies much of the time. I mean, our bodies are there, stretched out on the couch, the heat of the MacBook warming our lap – but it's all happening in our heads. Everything else is numbed.

An hour of yoga a day brings you back to your body. Not only that, you tune in and become aware of what seems like *another* body in your own body. This other body is complex and subtle: one side moves more easily than the other; some days it's all-powerful, other days there's no juice in the tank; some days are full of energy, other times you just want to stretch out and rest. In yoga, where awareness is drawn everywhere – even to the breath – this disassociation falls away. At least, that's what it's like for me. And yoga and meditation have been effective in fighting this disassociation. In short, they make me feel more alive, even if feeling more alive means feeling more pain, sadness, loss and anxiety – and, yes, also during the six weeks, joy. And that's a good thing.

Adam Whiting says there are two ways to look at modern yoga practice:

> One, the entry point, the surface level – people moving their bodies and stretching for an hour a day. Just this physical output of energy is benefiting them on a physical level. Their hips are getting more open, they're no longer experiencing back pain, they are feeling healthier, and this helps with wellness.
>
> Then there is a subtle energy in the postures. A skilled teacher can create a specific sequence combining the postures with specific breath techniques that can create a profound change on an energetic level. Beyond the surface of a stronger, more open, more supple body is an ocean of energetic channels. Sure, some of it has these mystical, magical undertones, but these techniques are not mysticism or witchcraft – it's science.

⁂

Friday is the last official night of the project and we do a really tough groove class with Adam and all these loquacious models who have not been part of the Modern Yogi Project – or maybe they once were, but have now graduated to full, proper yogis. They greet each other with kisses at the start of the class and keep high-fiving each other and doing handstands. At the end of the ninety minutes, Adam gets out his guitar and sings Whitney Houston's 'I Want to Dance with Somebody' as we are lying there drenched in our own sweat. It's a cappella, full of yearning, and unexpectedly moving and beautiful.

Then, when the song is over, we all sit in a semicircle and do three long *omms* in rounds. They seem to run over each other and through me and last for a long time, mingling with a kind of after-glow of the classical guitar chords, like a bath of sound, and I think that this is the right note to end on – literally.

But after class there is a graduation party of sorts and the yogi girls sit around eating nori rolls and talking about bad Tinder dates. I don't stay long; instead I get an Uber to a dinner party in Bronte and I notice one of the guests – a director – has brought his own food, wrapped in foil. I pour some champagne and wonder if he's gluten-free and maybe brought his own meal – which would be sad, but very much of the times, so I don't say anything.

Later I am relieved to find it is not gluten-free, it's actually a large hash cake and we all eat it before dinner and everything is hilarious and there is good linen and shiny tableware and steaming bowls of curry and crisp wine and I can't stop laughing and then I think, *The modern yogi course wasn't supposed to end like this.* But of course it was always going to end like this. This is my path – what C.S. Lewis calls a 'secret road' that we are all on, but each road is different. I like to think that I'm walking in the middle of the road, between the wellness lane and the hedonism lane, trying not to get run over by cars. Maybe I am meant to pick a side. But right now, I can't – and that's okay.

**

In January of 2016 a Los Angeles jury ordered my old mate Bikram Choudhury to pay $6.4 million in punitive damages to his former legal adviser, Minakshi Jafa-Bodden. Jafa-Bodden had initially sued (and won over $900,000) for sexual harassment, gender discrimination and wrongful termination.

Bikram claimed during the trial that he had run out of money – although on further questioning he admitted to owning a fleet of more than forty luxury cars. He said he had donated all the vehicles to the government to found the 'Bikram auto engineering school for children'. According to Jezebel, a spokesperson for the government said, essentially, 'Lol no.' If I could talk to Bikram now I would say two things to him. One: you were right – if you do yoga every day you will get lean and look good. And two: you are a total dick.

**

Winter has turned into spring – and I don't do yoga at the moment. The anxiety has gone too, thank God. It left as mysteriously as it arrived. One day I just noticed I felt 'normal'. The sick feeling in the pit of my stomach was gone. I never get to the bottom of why it appeared in the first place when I was so intensely engaged in a practice that was meant to chill me out. The New-Age, witchy part of me thinks – and I have no evidence for this – that when we radically try to shake something up (suddenly start doing lots of exercise, or lots of meditation, or eating differently) our more subtle energy system can be thrown. It can put up a firewall in protest at all the change, like a low hum of anxiety, or it can become fatigued. The body and all its workings seem at times more mysterious to me than distant galaxies and other planets.

What else? After months of paperwork, and negotiating with banks, I bought that little cottage in the country in a place without yoga studios or juice bars. Now, at night, all I can hear are the frogs in the creek and, in the morning, the magpies. I go to the gym five days a week and do weights, supervised by a really muscly guy called Lionel who doesn't say much but sometimes surprises me with passionate outbursts when I am doing split squats: 'Strong Brigid! Strong Brigid!' he'll say, which makes me look up, then wobble and lose my balance. Rihanna blasts from the speakers and I lie facedown on some machine and do single leg curls, and all I think about is the count of reps. I'm bored. Of course I'm bored – but after the tumult of winter, that's fine. It all works if you do it often enough, all the yoga and the running and the weights. After all, it's just moving your body, and that is what we are meant to do.

But with yoga there's something else, something other than movement, some other alchemy which gets all of us – teachers, students, celebrities and beginners – in its thrall. There's something else at work, other than the contraction and release of muscle, other than your heart pumping your blood a bit harder.

Yoga opens you up. Channels within you that you didn't know you had (the body within your body) make themselves felt. These channels force you open and make you feel more loose and alive.

The yoga sermons lose their potential to annoy and instead can hit you in tender, devastating places.

You drink them up. You didn't realise you were so thirsty.

SERENE

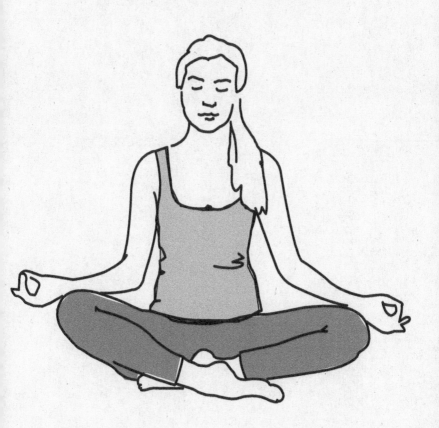

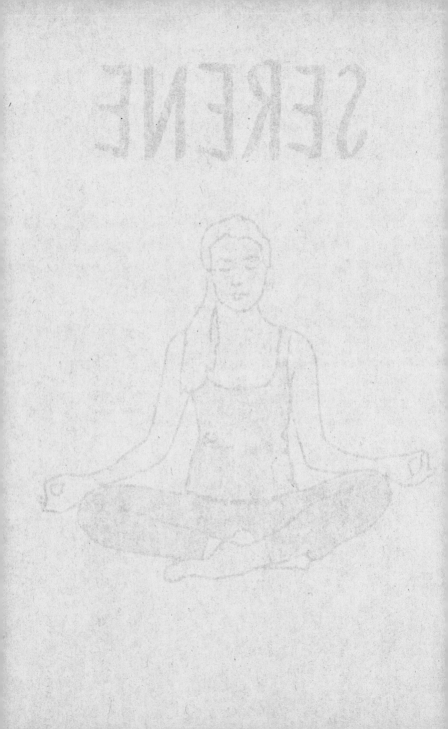

t's a mild winter in Western Australia. Patches of wildflowers have already blossomed, and the road weaves through the canola fields like a ribbon in bright yellow hair. I'm in the car with my three younger brothers, and we are driving to the monastery town of New Norcia, where they will drop me off to do a religious retreat. It's my first, if you don't count the ones we had to do for school, and I am nervous.

The week before, I had hopped jauntily on a bus at Sydney's Central Station for a travel assignment and disembarked in Perth five days later, bent over like a crone. The five-day trip across the Nullarbor had soldered my body into the shape of the seat on the Greyhound bus. We'd driven through each night and emerged from the darkness into brilliant dawns and then ... nothing. The road was flat and featureless. Kangaroos moved around the periphery like the dots that swim in your vision when you're tired. There were two drivers and they did the trip in shifts. On the bus were just four other passengers. We all sat apart and didn't make eye contact, even at the roadhouses and toilet blocks. To start a conversation might get you caught in something dull for days, duller even than the road. It was a bitch of an assignment – sleeping sitting up, truck-stop pies for dinner, and, at the end, the gleaming Perth bus depot, rinsed with morning sun.

The travel editor of my newspaper knew the assignment would be gruelling and not particularly glamorous. Would I perhaps like to do another travel story when I arrived in Perth? Cover something I was truly interested in? Maybe Rottnest Island? Or the Margaret River wineries?

'Well, there is this place,' I tell him. 'It's sort of weird. A hippy I met at a fruit market told me about it. It's a Benedictine monastery in the middle of nowhere and they accept guests.'

'Odd place to choose, but yeah, sure,' said my editor. 'Whatever floats your boat.'

And so off I went.

*

That year, 2005, I'd started having this weird *thing* with spirituality and religion, a tentative flirtation that seemed to come from nowhere. In those early days, I couldn't quite own up to it, and was disguising my curiosity under the detachment of reporting assignments for the *Sydney Morning Herald*.

Initially I started attending evangelical church services as a reporter. For youth night after work on a Friday or for service on a Sunday, I trekked ninety minutes out to the suburbs and the mega-church Hillsong. I was fascinated with this new, different and spectacular way people were worshipping. It was such a break from the traditional church of my youth – the cycle of sitting, kneeling and standing, the murmured incantation of the Sanctus, the incense and the old men in purple vestments. The modern churches were fishers of men – just like religion has been forever, but on their hooks was a tastier type of bait. They knew how people were living – these aspirational, prosperous John Howard voters in the suburbs – so when there was a group baptism at the church, there was also a giant screen showing rugby league, with a free sausage sizzle. The church leaders I interviewed spoke as if religion were a product: was it attractive enough, did it offer enough for people to *choose* it? Self-realisation and self-actualisation were recurring themes in our discussions.

I found myself being drawn in. I was living the high life in Sydney. I had a good newspaper job and a flat in Potts Point with my friend Patrick, a political staffer. We fancied ourselves as It kids, part of a scene where everyone seemed to work in politics or the media. We hosted a lot of dinner parties and on some perfect, rowdy nights in our cave-like flat, it felt like we were at the centre of the universe.

But what I was really seeking under the noise, movement and entertainment of my life was something deeper, more quiet and difficult to fathom. It was a quicksilver element that moved beneath the surface of all things. In this mysterious, non-secular space, things existed that could be felt but not seen.

Something else also existed there: serenity. I define this not just as walking around feeling chilled, but, in the words of a religious friend of mine, as 'the peace that the world cannot give'.

I didn't have serenity at home or at work – there was too much noise and excitement. I had to look for it, but I wasn't sure where. Did it exist out there – at a yoga retreat? Or a church? Or was it in you, in some hard-to-reach place that only the mystics and the saints could access? And, if so, how could a normal schlub like me get there? (This question about whether serenity and divinity can be drawn from an external source, such as church-based worship, or whether divinity resides within, is one of the perennial debates in religious/spiritual circles.)

Serenity was the missing piece of the puzzle in my quest for wellness. I had been doing yoga for around six years but hadn't started connecting with the spiritual stuff it offered. Time and time again, year after year after year, I would be told: you can get the clean, lean body, you can glow on the outside, but unless you attend to your inner life, the project is only partly complete. The balance is off. Serenity is the rock on which all else can be built. If your foundations are built on sand, then all that rests on them is liable to collapse.

And so, in 2005, in Western Australia, I began the search for serenity. It would prove infinitely more difficult and ultimately more rewarding than my quest to be clean and lean. It would take me to all corners of the globe, and expose me to many of the world's major religions, including Christianity, Hinduism, Islam and Buddhism. It would also introduce me to many people who had stripped the major religions for parts, and constructed something new, modern and strange. 'This is how you get serenity,' they would say, serving you food with complicated rituals and rules attached (food that had been dried and then cooked at temperatures of less than 46 degrees, or prepared by people wearing only white garments, or farmed in accordance with the ancient principles of the terroir), making you meditate on earth that contained electromagnetic vibrations or listen to ancient Sanskrit poetry – and charging you thousands for it.

Sometimes it would work . . . a little bit of this, a little bit of that. But some of these 'products', as I would come to think of them, were a scam – latching on to what is a very human, and sometimes very desperate urge to glimpse the divine and also find inner peace.

I wasn't the only one looking. The search for serenity was becoming big business in the wellness industry, and over the next twelve years I would see it morph from a fringe, hippy concern to something vast, global and corporate.

Serenity itself, *the peace that the world cannot give*, is a slippery beast. I'd find it, and hang on for dear life, but if I didn't pay attention, if I didn't create rituals and habits around it, it would vanish, and I would be in the same stressed, agitated place I had started. That feeling of something solid, immoveable and grounded was missing.

But first, the start ...

New Norcia is a remote Benedictine monastery town almost two hours from the most isolated city in the world – Perth. This makes New Norcia one of the most far-flung retreats on the planet. In the middle of nowhere, there won't be any distractions. Perfect, right? Travel writer Pico Iyer, who regularly attends retreats, spoke highly of his visit to New Norcia:

> In the thirty years of almost constantly travelling around the world, I have seldom met a place so clarifying and calm as New Norcia. It makes you think again about what matters; it returns you to a sense of stillness and community that's hard to find in the modern world; it refreshes the soul better than any holiday. The only hardship of coming here is leaving.

It's also a hardship to get there. But otherwise there are few barriers to entry. You just contact the monastery and reserve a room. You don't need to be religious, and there's a suggested donation for food and accommodation that is quite affordable (around eighty dollars a night). It fits with the Benedictine creed: *Welcome the stranger as you would welcome Christ himself*.

'Please come with me,' I beg my brothers as we near the unusual-looking township of New Norcia. We've been playing pool and drinking beer in the old, grand and shady pub at the edge of town. It was nice in there, convivial and social, even though I was beaten at pool. The four of us – my three brothers and me – are hardly ever together all at once. Why am I cutting short time with them to spend time with *me*? After all, I'm with me all the time.

I am losing signal on my phone one bar at a time, and my heart sinks as my brothers drop me at the gates. There's no TV at the monastery – that's fine, but I've become addicted to season five of *Big Brother* and no one will be able to text me the winner. The lack of comms and the strange old-fashioned buildings make me nervous, like Marty McFly finding himself in 1955.

New Norcia is unlike any place I've visited in Australia. Fringed with palm trees and surrounded by fields of wheat, it could have been lifted straight from the plains of Spain's Andalusia. It's incongruous, plonked here in Western Australian farming country. It has two now-abandoned orphanages, once used to house children who were not strictly orphans – they were Indigenous kids, some taken from their families under government order (though I had to really prise anything about the stolen generation out of the guide when I went on a town tour).

In 2017 the town made news for having the highest rate of clerical sexual abuse allegations for any Catholic institution or diocese, according to figures released by the Royal Commission into Institutional Responses to Child Sexual Abuse. The report found 7 per cent of priests from all Catholic Church authorities across Australia were accused of child sexual abuse from 1950 to 2010, but for the Benedictine Community of New Norcia the number was more than triple that, at 21.5 per cent.

It's no surprise, then, that the town pulses with dark undercurrents – or, as one of my brothers observed just before he shut the car door and drove away, 'This place has bad vibes.'

There have been no abuse allegations since 1980, and the town has reinvented itself as a tourist destination and gourmet food producer. According to the tour guide, the Benedictine monks make some of the most sought-after bread in the state, served at many of Perth's top restaurants. From the New Norcia gift shop you can also purchase olive oil, something delicious and very calorific called New Norcia nut cake, pan chocolatti, almond biscotti, wine, port and beer.

But beyond the pub and the gift shop, the monastery itself is vast and foreboding, set on 8000 hectares of farmland. It's the sort of place you go alone, to be alone. The tourism is of the spiritual variety. There, you look for God, serenity – whatever you want to call it – and you work things out. One guest tells me that men turn up here in the middle of the night, having driven from Perth – desperate, with nowhere else to go. As per the Benedictine creed, the monks take them in, feed and water them, and in return the men work on the farm. In the silence and the space they get their heads together over three, four, six months. It's like something from a Tim Winton novel. One day in the dining room my eyes lock with a young man in work boots with a missing thumb and a radiant sadness. He could have been a template for one of Winton's broken men.

The monastery is home to a community of sixteen monks who follow the rules laid down by Saint Benedict, the father of Western monasticism. Benedict (480–543) was a young Roman ascetic who wanted to devote himself to spiritual exercises and communal living, emulating the Egyptian Desert Fathers and Mothers of the third century. He wrote a handbook on how to live monastically, including the rule that monks should take a vow of obedience, stability and communal living to a particular abbey, where they would spend the rest of their lives. That's right – the rest of their lives! It is so rare these days for anyone to spend their life doing one thing, in one place. Modern spiritual life – including retreats – tends to have more of a 'drop-in' quality. You have an intense few days or a week in a place, then go back to your normal life. The idea of committing to a lifelong spiritual practice in one place is mind-bending.

The monks spend their time mostly in prayer, observing the following timetable: 5.15am – Vigils, 6.45am – Lauds, 7.30am – Conventual Mass, 12.05pm – Midday Prayer, 2.30pm – Afternoon Prayer, 6.30pm – Vespers, 8.15pm – Complines. The rest of the day is taken up by two hours' work in the morning, two hours' work in the afternoon, one hour of communal conversation (the day is mainly spent in silence), and meals, eaten in silence with someone reading aloud from a book.

Immediately I chafe at one of the rules – male guests are allowed to eat with the monks, but the female guests must eat in the general dining room. This seems like such a throwback until

I remember where I am: *a Benedictine monastery in the middle of nowhere*. It's not meant to be progressive.

On the first night in the general dining hall, I share meals with two women in their sixties. I begin a conversation full of steam, only to be greeted with pursed lips, cross looks and silence. One woman points to the hand-drawn sticker on her jumper. It reads, 'Hello my name is Jan & I am on silent retreat.'

'Oh, hullo, Jan. Does that mean you're not talking?' I ask idiotically. I am answered, again, with silence.

The silence at New Norcia is famous. People come here from all round the world to hear ... nothing. They just want to luxuriate in the great, vast, heavy silence of the place. In this context, small talk at dinner is a pollutant.

Serenity is reached at New Norcia via silence, prayer and routine. The prayer timetable is pinned up in the dining room. Guests are encouraged to join the monks for prayer and mass daily at 7:30am. Most guests attend all prayer services – and then when the monks go back to the farm, the bakery or olive press, guests usually rest, read, contemplate or meditate or ramble around the massive farm. Apart from meals there's very little interaction with others at the monastery.

I speak with one of the monks, who tells me one of the most important elements of staying at New Norcia is developing a closer relationship with God. Strip away noise, entertainment, mobile phone reception and shopping, and replace it with farming, country life and daily prayer, and 'the spiritual communication channels open up'.

Some people go on retreats so they can find God, but the Benedictine way is to assume that God is already there; it's just a matter of opening yourself up to him. It's harder to open yourself up to God if you are talking all the time – to others or in the endless, mostly tedious monologues we have in our heads. The silence, in this context, has a sort of preparatory quality: you prepare yourself to be passive, to yield, to receive and accept. The intellect and the ego must recede for this to happen.

At New Norcia, it's easy to feel as though God – or at least some spiritual presence – exists. You're stripped of distractions. No phone signal, no TV. At night the sky is vast, black and thick with stars. Apart from the pub, there are no buildings nearby, so no light pollution. The darkness is complete and the clean, dry air has a purity about it, smelling of nothing but the faint, sweet taint of wheat. There's the occasional rumble from a truck or car travelling down the Great Northern Highway, the rustle of the wind through the high, dry grass, and the bells for prayers, but otherwise it's totally and utterly quiet.

I go for walks around the farm at night after Complines (it's so dark that one night I fall in a hole) and register the vastness of the sky and the low clouds and moon as a distinct, almost malevolent physical presence (aka the 'bad vibes'). The silence and the emptiness have an oppressive, blanket-like quality and do not, for me, equate with peace. Instead they leave me feeling unsettled and agitated. After several days of this – plus prayers – I am keen to leave. Some of the prayers are disquieting, Old Testamenty stuff. We are warned of this with flyers at breakfast, informing us that today we would be reciting some 'problem psalms'. It's like a monastic trigger warning.

That week, I experience New Norcia as a sort of shadow land. God (or something) is here – I sense a mysterious presence – but it's not a calming sort of god. It is large and awesome, and, when I'm walking under that massive sky, in a curious inversion of my *Big Brother* addiction, I feel watched.

At least I'll sleep well here, it's so quiet! I think on my first night as I turn in early in my little room near the chapel. But no! New Norcia has other plans for me. That night I have nightmares of epic proportions: visceral and squalid, more real and scary than anything I've experienced before (apart from the time I took acid, had too much and my hand disappeared). It's still dark when the bells for Vigils wake me at 5am, and it's only after Vespers at 6:30pm that I stop feeling frightened. The nightmares also leave a curious moral taint, like my subconscious is throwing up things I've previously locked away: anyone I've ever sold out, everyone who's sold me out, every story I've ever written that someone didn't like, every bit of shade thrown my way, all the gossip, all the shame, all the insecurities.

The next night I dream that all my teeth are falling out in shards, and I try but fail to push them back into my gums. It's terrifying and grotesque. When I'm woken for Vigils, the first thing I do is check my mouth, unable to shake off images of blood, saliva and enamel crumbling like broken biscuits into my hands. That evening in the courtyard, agitated and distracted, I risk censure for breaking the silence and approach someone who turns out to be a lovely and quite chatty theology student visiting from Kentucky. 'This is not a place you go to lightly,' he said of New Norcia (not the courtyard). 'This place kinda stirs things up in you. I've had nightmares as well. It has a vibe to it.'

'Did your teeth fall out?'

'Pardon?'

'In your dream.'

'Err, no, they didn't, ma'am.'

I meet a few more young people later that week. They come as a group every year and make an odd trio in Vespers – wearing beanies, they read from their psalm sheets then adjourn for ciggies in the courtyard.

Another guy, in his twenties with a thin, sharp face that makes him look much younger, tells me he's been coming to the monastery regularly for several years after beating a drug addiction back in Perth. His life was out of control and home detox was a nightmare but ultimately worked. Going to the monastery for the first time was important, as it 'broke a pattern inside me', he says. Whenever he comes, he resets his commitment to being clean. He suggests that my nightmares could just be an adjustment I have to make. Like a junkie having withdrawals, I am detoxing from the trash of modern life.

He also tells me he doesn't know what's happening in the *Big Brother* house, if Tim is still in there and if one or both of the Logan twins have been evicted (one of the twins, Logan Greg, would go on to win the series). In my spare time I walk around the higher ground of the town, arm aloft with my Nokia brick, hoping for a phone signal, but my prayers remain unanswered.

At New Norcia I don't find the serenity I'm searching for. Instead, I get the opposite experience: turmoil. I suspect if I had stayed at the retreat longer I would have come out the other end fine – peaceful, having sorted through the mess in my mind. Maybe the bad dreams were the first part of this sorting process – like my brain was throwing up the trash first, tilling the soil to prepare for something new. I just didn't give it enough time.

The silence does allow me to see that there is a lot of disquiet in my subconscious. It is like going into an attic filled with junk that hasn't been touched for years. By moving a few things around, lifting things up, inspecting them, the surface is upset, dust and dirt fly about, bats are disturbed and flap around – and you just want to shut the door, pretend the whole thing didn't happen. But it has happened. The right thing to do is finish what I've started, no matter how painful the process. I feel like this acknowledge-ment is the first step on the path to serenity – a path I realise now is more difficult than first thought. After all, people spend their whole lives in the monastery – serenity is a project that has to be made anew each day.

The thing that was missing for me at New Norcia was the les-sons. I went in cold, and you don't just stumble across serenity. You have to be shown the map and taught how to drive yourself there. Then you have to work at it again and again and again.

Back in Sydney, in the taxi on the way home from the air-port, past the bright lights, the madness and noise of Kings Cross, there's breaking news on the radio. London's been attacked by ter-rorists – scores dead, hundreds maimed. The cabbie swears softly and turns up the volume. We drive slowly past the Coke sign and the neon-lit strip clubs because drunk people keep staggering in front of the cab. I think of the rustle of the long, dry grass in the night winds and the monks praying out there in the vast West Australian silence, oblivious to what's going on in the wider world, and that T.S. Eliot line comes unbidden: *Lips that would kiss/ Form prayers to broken stone*.

A year later I'm living in London, just round the corner from where the bombs went off. I'm working at CNN as a features writer, which to this day remains one of the great jobs of my life. I'm plunged into the expensive, scented, pampered, posh segment of the wellness industry, where you pay people to touch you. My job is to review day spas. Two colleagues and I are working on a mini health and wellness website. We gather for editorial meetings and discuss our ideas.

'Yar, I think we should do veganism. There are all these celeb vegans around at the moment – like Stella McCartney.'

'Yar, great! You should go vegan for a week. "My Vegan Hell", or some shit like that. What else we got?'

'Bespoke barber shops for men – the ones that serve Veuve and have heated towels.'

'Yar, fab!'

'There's this spa in Mayfair – they do birdshit facials. Apparently the phosphate in the shit is great for your skin!'

'Love it! There's also the five-hour gold-leaf spa thingy treatment at the Mandarin Oriental in Knightsbridge. They roll you in *real* gold leaf and then baste you in a private sauna.'

'I think that's where the reflexology guy is. The one who used to work on Princess Diana.'

'He also did Mandela's feet.'

And on it goes. All the spas open their doors to us – and from limb to limb we are stroked on a daily basis by London's finest.

My housemates have serious jobs on newspapers – foreign desk at the *Telegraph*, business desk at the *Times*. They are pasty from the lack of sun, their necks and shoulders aching from hours spent hunched in front of computers under fluorescent lights. When they come home from work, shattered, I'm lying on the couch, glistening and dewy, sleepy and slippery from all the treatments, oils and creams that have been slathered on me. The therapists instruct me not to shower after the treatments so the lotions can soak in. I'm so moisturised that my grip is terrible. I can barely open doors. Yet I always smell expensive – like a wallet full of flowers. My main concern in life is that my skeletal structure might dissolve because I'm being massaged so much.

Then one week at our regular Soho House meetings ('Who wants to volunteer for the coffee bean facial? We also need to cover the Holborn Musical Massage.') the topic of meditation comes up. Meditation … wot dat? Some old-timey thing practised by Beatles in India and rich hippies in Hampstead? But who does it now? Who has the time or the patience – particularly *right now*, with the internet and this Facebook thing suddenly everywhere, taking up everyone's time?

Mindfulness will become mainstream about seven years later, in 2014, a resurgence caused partly by the internet itself, which will splinter and shatter everyone's concentration into teeny-tiny shards. But in 2007, meditation is still mysterious, even kind of daggy, associated with joss sticks and ugly clothing made from hemp.

My editor dispatches me to the London Buddhist Centre in Bethnal Green to find out more. Maybe meditation is the thing that was missing during my time at New Norcia. Maybe it would give me the skills to stop, go inward and find serenity in a structured, deliberate way. You see, despite my great job, moisturised skin and relaxed muscles, a hunger still niggles away at me. A hunger of the spiritual kind. It's never really gone away. I think of it as something submerged (like I'd been the week before, in a skin-plumping rose-petal bubble bath at Jurlique in Chiswick).

Over the English summer I'd stayed at a monastery in Wales for a week, and one lonely Christmas during my first months in London I'd stopped at a church in Bloomsbury after passing by and hearing a soaring fragment of a hymn. In a cold pew down the back I softly wept for reasons I did not understand. Something was missing.

After work one Thursday night I go to the London Buddhist Centre, meet Maitreyabandhu – he has one name, like Prince – and learn how to meditate. In one of the centre's rooms, with the lights low, I practise something called Loving Kindness meditation with a group of people, mostly in their twenties and thirties, from all over the city. It feels like sending ripples of goodness into the world using only the power of our thoughts. Maitreyabandhu, the Buddhist monk who teaches us, is convinced that meditation is an effective treatment for people with anxiety and depression, and is building a new hall in the centre to cater for this cohort.

He is ahead of his time. He sees meditation as not just a tried-and-true way of relaxing, but also a bulwark against the distractions that are multiplying at a rate never experienced by humans before (this is around the time that Apple releases the first-ever iPhone, and everything changes). Distraction is the enemy of serenity. Serenity is depths and silence. Distraction is surfaces and noise. Aldous Huxley wrote of his famous novel, *Brave New World*, 'Non-stop distractions of the most fascinating nature are deliberately used as instruments of policy, for the purpose of preventing people from paying too much attention to the realities of the social and political situation.' And to this we could add paying too much attention to our quiet, inner, spiritual life. Man's appetite for distraction, writes Huxley, is 'almost infinite'. He was writing from the relative calm of the pre-internet 20th century, a time of 'news-papers and television', about distractions that 'exceeded even the greatest excesses of Rome'. What would he make of today, when distractions are so numerous and overpowering they exceed even the visions of his brilliant imagination?

After the meditation class finishes – and I feel more relaxed than if I'd just had a three-hour, four-hand massage in a replica Egyptian crypt in a Kensington day spa – Maitreyabandhu explains to me why meditation is more necessary now than ever: 'Modern life is incredibly complicated and fast. That is very stressful for the mind and body, and people's quality of life diminishes. We are obsessed with choice, and people often choose things that are not in their long-term interests. You can easily feel you've taken the wrong path.'

I confess to him that for the last couple of years I've been a secret searcher – looking for something without pinning down exactly what it is that I'm looking for. Maitreyabandhu sees it all the time. 'People feel there's a definite meaning vacuum,' he tells me. 'People are increasingly realising materialism is not working; choice is not working. The basic assumption is that the more choice you have, the happier you'll be. But what people really need is a sense that their lives matter.' As a result of our rushed lives we can also lose touch with ourselves. Meditation is a way of checking in and assessing how things are going. We may be able to catch situations or patterns before they develop into something more entrenched.

What Maitreyabandhu says makes a lot of sense. Rather than just treating stress with an expensive massage, a practice like meditation tackles the stress before it starts to build up. From a place of calm and serenity we can better tackle the vicissitudes of life. That night I sign up for a week-long 'urban retreat' that Maitreyabandhu is running, to see if meditating every day and being mindful can improve my moods, sleep patterns and anxiety levels.

Before it starts, I meet with the other participants. Each person has a different reason for wanting to practise meditation. Some people want to eat more mindfully and cook more, others want to go out less and have a few more quiet nights at home reading a book. One man didn't want to lose his temper so much with his builders, another wants to reduce the importance of his work and have a more balanced life.

If there's one common issue in this group, it's anger triggered by commuting on public transport. Everyone starts the day in a bad mood as a result. 'It all goes downhill from there,' said one Tube-hater. Many also report being anxious or worried about the future and are not inclined to 'live in the moment'. These are all concerns common to anyone living in a large and busy city. But could we stay in London and still find serenity?

Maitreyabandhu advises us to keep our urban retreat week goals realistic. Things like meditating at the London Buddhist Centre for an hour before work are well and good, he advised, but if you are an hour and a half from the centre, are you really likely to rise at 4am each day, particularly if public transport makes you angry? Won't that make you more unhappy, and defeat the purpose?

Instead he says to aim to come into the centre and meditate for just one or two mornings this week. And instead of radically changing habits such as diet, do something like switch off the TV for a week, or walk to work.

What is important about the week is to be what Maitreyabandhu calls 'mindful'. Mindfulness is a technique that can lead you to serenity. It is the first time I've heard the word that by 2014 would be here, there and everywhere – used as a cure-all for everything, from becoming more productive to having better sex to making more money. It would even be so ubiquitous in the corporate world that some charge the practice with enforcing the neoliberal agenda. Corporations like mindfulness because it 'keeps us within the fences of the neoliberal capitalist paradigm', management professor and Zen practitioner Ronald Purser says in the *New Yorker*. 'It's saying, "It's your problem, get with the program, fix your stress, and get back to work!"' But all that is to come. In 2007, mindfulness has yet to be corrupted by the market.

Maitreyabandhu explains that mindfulness involves being present in the moment, being aware of your surroundings and not letting your mind constantly race ahead to what may happen in the future or dwell excessively on what happened in the past. He advises that mindfulness can be achieved by spending time away from the internet and TV, walking instead of driving, and, of course, meditating.

While we will be spending time at work and doing our usual routine during the retreat, it will be with a twist – with this twist promoting mindfulness. Maitreyabandhu will be sending us text messages throughout the week, and we can also log on to his daily blog. Maitreyabandhu advises us to put a shrine on our desks and change our computer passwords to something that will remind us we're on retreat. We are given a green wristband to wear throughout the week. Each time we look at it we are supposed to remember we are on retreat and to be mindful. Someone suggests that whenever we hear a siren – a very London sound, particularly for me as I live near a major hospital – we should remember to be mindful.

Maitreyabandhu also allocates us a retreat buddy. He advises us to identify potential stress points in the week, such as a deadline or a meeting with someone we find difficult, and contact our buddy to help us remain calm.

It's Monday morning, the first day of the urban retreat, and the first text from Maitreyabandhu arrives. *Relax your eyes, relax your belly*, it reads. I am on a bus, stuck in Oxford Street traffic, and suddenly I feel relaxed and mindful. I puff my stomach out, I slouch in my seat and touch the green wristband. I'm not just on a packed bus going to work, I'm on retreat.

Feel the sun on your back! he texts as I am walking down Great Marlborough Street – and as instructed, I do. It feels good.

It is a gentler introduction to the workings of your inner life than going into a monastery cold, like I'd done with New Norcia. And because you are still working and living in your city while doing the retreat, it follows that the things you learn can be integrated more fully into your normal life.

The week continues. I go to work. I go to the gym. I go to the theatre. I go to the pub. I spend at least twelve hours in the spas of west London, being rubbed down with salmon roe foam or chocolate mousse or fox placenta. I have a flotation tank session. I have a whole body scrub exfoliant thing. I have a jet massage thing. I have a hot stone thing. I have an oil scalp massage. I lie in dim waiting areas on chaise longues in hotel bathrobes, sipping lemongrass tea from tiny ceramic cups and reading *Tatler* in cool blue rooms where it's forever twilight. It's lovely but I can now see this is all surface serenity. The real stuff lies within and cannot be bought or sold.

While I'm doing the same things I always do, the text messages and the blog keep me focused on being on retreat. I become more aware of what stresses me out, so I do pre-emptive strikes. I walk to work instead of taking public transport. When I go to the pub I have one drink instead of three or four (conscious drinking, it's called) and I spend a couple of nights at home, cooking healthy food.

The highlight of the urban retreat is when I haul myself out of bed before 6am and go to the Buddhist Centre for 7am group meditation. It is tough. I am still new to meditation and an hour sitting in silence feels like having an itch I can't scratch. Time moves so *slowly*. But afterwards I feel energised. Before we head off to our various workplaces, the group has breakfast together at the cafe next door, all of us still wearing our green wristbands. There's a sense of community developing. It feels good.

Maitreyabandhu warns that discipline is needed in order to continue to experience this meditator's high. 'One of the big disciplines in life is to put aside time for things that are good for you. We've all watched hours of TV and felt empty. How do we convince ourselves to do something better?'

I leave the retreat vowing to meditate every day. Such good intentions! But life and its many distractions get in the way – and Bethnal Green requires three line changes on the Tube and a bus. It's not meant to be – at least not this time. The techniques I was learning are harder to integrate into my real life than I thought. My job is busy, I'm making lots of new friends, London is exciting and on weekends I get the Eurostar to Paris, or take four days off in Italy. I am young and have few cares. I start working on a novel, and go inward that way – via my imagination. Serenity can wait. At this point in my life, I feel I don't really need it after all.

But, of course, life changes – it always does.

By 2010 I have returned to Australia, and superficially my life resembles the life I had before I left for London, when I was working at the *Sydney Morning Herald* and living in Potts Point. Sydney is a beautiful trashbag who won't let me go too deep or get too much sleep. I play hard and work hard. Serenity is not a priority. My new job is as a news editor of a tabloid news website. My shifts often start at 5am. I am running on what we call the Tabloid Treadmill. It never lets up.

Warm, windy dawns; wet, empty streets; the occasional ghostly jogger running down New South Head Road in the dark; ABC News Radio on in the cab, with its urgent-seeming headlines repeated in fifteen-minute loops; weary, lonely taxi drivers ... By the time I get into work, I'm plugged into the vast matrix of news – the restless, relentless 24/7 newsgathering cycle that never sleeps. By 6am the team has read every major news website in the English-speaking world and I'm preparing the morning lists and commissions.

Information flows through me in an exhaustive and exhausting stream. When asked at the end of the day what stories we have done, I often can't remember. Synapses in my brain are blowing like small fuses connected to a faulty main that services a large city – I have zero short-term recall. The London years of massages and facials and mid-morning editorial meetings at Soho House over toasted ciabatta and jam are now like a dream. Maitreyabandhu and those cosy nights at the Buddhist Centre that made so much sense at the time also seem very far away.

But our website is the most read site in Australia. Based on the traffic, readers like stories about: brides, brides in peril, bad bridal wear, tattoos gone wrong, Photoshop gone wrong, plus-sized models, crime (particularly gruesome crimes), people killed or maimed by claw hammers, Josef Fritzl, people locked in dungeons, freaky animals, funny viral videos, Australian television celebrities, celebrities who have died.

It's crazy and I love it, but that same old ghost haunts the margins. The ghost who tells me it is not sustainable to live like this – drinks that finish at 1am, the early alarms, falling asleep while getting a pedicure and also – improbably – while getting my legs waxed. At least one full day each weekend is spent sleeping. Daytime sleeps are heavy, long and dreamless, like mini comas.

Then there are all the large lattes, the cups piling up on my desk in a curdling tower, all the stodgy food-court lunches, all the sweet, tangy gulps of sauvignon blanc in the Sydney sun and the cadged cigarettes in the open-air bar downstairs, all the dawn taxis and the urgent music that precedes the news bulletins. Urgency and adrenalin, our constant, never-sated lust for breaking news, for the next, the next, the next thing – it's like a blowtorch to serenity.

I can feel myself burning out. I need some reprieve from this pace, and to reconnect with meditation. It worked like a temporary miracle in London, but I haven't been able to summon the energy or the willpower to integrate it into my daily life. So I do that thing a lot of cashed-up Western women do when they feel stressed out: go online, google 'yoga retreat' and bang in their credit card details. The retreat I choose is in Sri Lanka. Britain's *Observer* has called it the 'best yoga retreat in the world', and it promises a more holistic approach to health and wellbeing, using ancient Ayurvedic medicine. Each guest has a consultation with an Ayurvedic doctor and a choice of treatments.

I fly into the capital, Colombo, to see my old college pal Brett, who works for the UN. He's been relocated there after many years in the north, and months of intense civil war conflict. His town had been shelled, and many of his friends and colleagues killed or injured. On the way to his place from the airport we drive past a massive structure, the top of its walls covered with rolls of barbed wire.

'That's the prison,' he says flatly. 'Some of my friends are in there, being tortured. Others have been disappeared.'

Welcome to Sri Lanka. Namaste.

Brett lives in a colonial pile in the centre of town that has an air of dilapidated glamour. The high life has come and gone. Tall, compound-like walls, large, musty bedrooms, trees growing through the lounge-room floor, monkeys overhead, cracks in the marble ... The jungle bashes down the door. I imagine previous generations of inhabitants as Somerset Maugham types – British civil servants gone to seed, the wild gardens running through their kitchens as they tried to negotiate railways, schools and the price of tea. But the streets of old Colombo are also thick with rats.

Brett emerges from his room the next morning red-eyed and shaken. I peer in. It looks like he got drunk and trashed it. A massive rat has crawled up through the plumbing in Brett's ensuite and chewed its way through the wood in the door. It ran at Brett and attacked him before he set at it with a cricket bat. Things are broken, bookshelves are turned over, furniture has been gnawed to bits. Just before dawn, Brett managed to push the rat back down the drain, placing a brick over it.

The next night the rat returns. It must be strong – somehow it manages to push aside the brick. Books and wood bear the marks of vicious little teeth. The rat has also shat everywhere.

I decide to get out of the house and explore Colombo in a tiny rickshaw decorated with plastic flowers and sequins. The driver, playing tour guide, takes me to his favourite beach, which is covered in rubbish and gloomy with pollution and light rain. After ninety seconds walking on the depressing beach, I step over a large plastic bag that is ripped and has stuff leaking out – like a corpse that has been stabbed and left to drain. I ask if I can sit back in the rickshaw.

'This is our best beach!'

'No, it's okay, I can see it from the rickshaw.'

'You should walk on the beach!'

'No, it's okay, I've seen enough.'

We have been walking together, which feels weirdly intimate. I don't even know him – I just flagged him down and sat in the back of his vehicle. Now we are like a couple, fighting, not holding hands, walking along an empty beach.

He sulks as I direct him to this place that sells really great salads, according to TripAdvisor. It's also a bookstore with a lot of post-colonial Sri Lankan and Indian literature – think Salman Rushdie and Arundhati Roy. I buy Eckhart Tolle's spiritual bestseller *The*

Power of Now to read on the yoga retreat – a move so cliched that I tell myself it's ironic.

I make my way to Ulpotha, a village deep in the interior of Sri Lanka that could have been dreamed up by some author in a magic-realist phase – Gabriel García Márquez, perhaps. I arrive at night and am given tea, then escorted by lamplight to my quarters. There is no electricity.

My room is a mud-brick hut with only one supporting wall, almost entirely open to the elements. A bed sits in the middle, covered by a tightly tucked-in mosquito net. Gas lamps glow low around the hut and a monkey runs past. The jungle at dusk suddenly fills with animal noises.

Ulpotha is a retreat and working village in central Sri Lanka, open to guests for part of the year. The backbone of the place is a community of villagers who have been in the area for generations. They live in similar huts to the guests', worship in the nearby temples, farm the land, cook the food and help run the retreat during the tourist season.

It's kind of like a farm stay mixed with an Ayurvedic health retreat mixed with the sort of luxe interiors that feature in *Condé Nast Traveller* – in the middle of Sri Lanka. And then there is the food – vegetarian and delicious, also prepared by the villagers. Without electricity, food is cooked over a fire. Breakfast is fresh bananas, unusual juices and coconut pancakes. There are pots of tea, made from leaves picked in the nearby farm. A villager is on hand with a machete if you want to open a fresh coconut to drink.

On my first day I'm walking through a carefully swept path in the jungle when I run into a bare-chested, middle-aged Englishman wearing a sarong.

'Careful of those monkeys,' he says, pointing up to branches thick with them. 'Yesterday I was having a shower and one of them nicked my watch!'

His name is Pete and he lives in Slough and works as a brick-layer. He's here with his wife, Sally, for two weeks and they are jumping out of their skins – vital with good health, their energy levels nuclear, their eyes bright, their faces and hair shiny. I look exactly as you would expect me to look: an unhealthy office worker who's had too much white wine, too much time online, and has just spent the last few days being terrified by a rat.

While I did want to look like my new friends from Slough, I wasn't sure if the Ayurvedic path was for me. Ayurvedic med-icine is one of the world's oldest holistic (whole-body) healing systems. The term 'Ayurveda' combines the Sanskrit words 'ayur' (life) and 'veda' (science or knowledge). Developed thou-sands of years ago in India, it is based on the belief that health and wellness depend on a delicate balance between the mind, body and spirit. Using these concepts, Ayurvedic physicians prescribe individualised treatments, including herbs and diet, exercise and lifestyle recommendations. It's still widely used in India and Sri Lanka today – sometimes in conjunction with Western medicine.

There are two categories of treatment available during my stay. There are the 'nice' treatments – preparatory things called oleation and fomentation therapies, including oil applications such as mas-sage, steam and medicinal bath therapies. Then there is the other sort, classified as 'elimination therapies'. These include enemas, bloodletting and vomiting (or 'purging', as it's delicately put in the retreat's literature).

Some of the oleation therapies involve searing yourself like a barramundi in a coffin-shaped cane basket, and prove to be uncomfortable. Or lathering yourself in oil like an early '80s porn star. I submit to a steam in one of the cane coffins but don't enjoy the experience. It feels like being in a primitive MRI.

Each guest, regardless of whether they sign up for an Ayurvedic program, gets a consultation with the retreat's doctor, Srilal Mudunkothge. He is an Ayurveda doctor of some renown, and I expect some esoteric Eastern wisdom. Instead he just looks me up and down, shrugs and says, 'Lay off the carbs after lunch.'

Easier said than done, mate. After breakfast one morning I cycle to the village clinic, where there are more than fifty locals crammed into the waiting room to see Dr Mudunkothge. So popular is the clinic that villagers sleep out overnight to get an appointment. The clinic dispenses free Ayurveda medicines in return for a symbolic offering of betel leaves.

In a sort of Robin Hood move, money to pay for this clinic comes from the yoga retreat, which is expensive – around $2000 a week. According to the Ulpotha clinic website, in its first ten years it treated over 15,000 patients and carried out over 47,000 consultations. The money raised from tourism also goes into keeping the village sustainable. The villagers use organic farming methods and ancient techniques such as threshing crops using buffalos.

This soothes my white guilt. Retreats in developing countries make me feel a little uneasy. Capitalism is a system so complete that it has swallowed up and repackaged even Eastern spirituality – and sells it back to us at Western prices. Retreats tap in to (or rip off or appropriate, depending on where you stand) ancient spiritual practices of the host country, but with the added bonus of having a lower cost base due to wage and infrastructure prices in that country. You certainly get more bang for your buck on retreat in Vietnam than you would in Byron Bay. But it's not just costs and cultural appropriation. There can also be a massive disconnect between the world of the retreat and the world outside the retreat. Sign up to a retreat and they'll usually offer to pick you up from the airport, not the city. The experience is more seamless, more magical, if you stay in the retreat bubble.

But I'm having fun in Ulpotha. Soon enough I forget my Sydney life – the early starts, the news cycle that spins so fast it's impossible to step back and read the patterns and the tea leaves, to get the big picture of what's really going on in the world. I forget all of that – and I forget the rat in Colombo, and Brett's stories of war and torture. I'm in the wellness bubble. I could stay here forever with Pete and Sally from Slough. With all the treatments we'll age backwards, just like Benjamin Button.

I get into the very healthy pattern of twice-daily yoga sessions in the gorgeous open pavilion that looks out over rice paddies. I'm going to yoga all the time because I have fallen for my yoga instructor. I love him! But I love him in the way you love your science teacher in Year 9: irrational, embarrassing afterwards. I experience his lessons as something romantic and meaningful – suffused with a kind of dreamy, slow-mo hot-buttered loveliness. A lock of sweaty Hugh Grant hair flops over his eye as he demonstrates revolved side angle pose. 'Yes, sir. Anything you want, sir.' This is the unspoken eros that can exist between student and teacher. He keeps me coming back to class.

At every mealtime, I seek out a seat beside him. There is a pattern here – I am always travelling to exotic locations and falling in lock step with diffident Englishmen. We'd meet for tea, walk around gardens, explore cities and exchange gifts, without anything actually happening – just a tender feeling between us, an enclosed sort of warmth. And when we'd part, there'd be a nostalgic afterglow, fading like a bruise. I would get these lovely romantic bruises time and time again, like I was a character stuck in a decades-long Merchant Ivory film, where the most erotic thing that happens is that the man touches the sleeve of the woman's dress for a beat longer than necessary.

I give him my Eckhart Tolle book, inscribed with a gushing message. But later, in yoga class, he drops me when he's trying to hold me aloft, demonstrating a pose. Perhaps I am too heavy and unwieldy (although he had no trouble picking up the couple from Slough). And just like that, the spell is broken.

But another spell takes its place – a discovery that is more intoxicating than a crush, partly, I suppose, because it is unexpected. It's the discovery of stillness. Finally! Stillness is the gateway to serenity. Serenity is like one of those wild animals that will only approach if you remain very still and quiet, like a statue. Yet we are so conditioned to recoil from stillness, confusing it with boredom or inertia. We don't really know how to do it. Before my breakthrough in Ulpotha, moments with nothing in them were to be rushed through. A stretch of quiet and inaction had no currency in my value system. Boredom was in the empty moments and boredom was to be avoided. I didn't know how deep and rich the experience of just sitting still could be, of looking – really looking – at something, particularly nature. Stillness made me uncomfortable in New Norcia and I was too excitable to be truly still in London. But in Sri Lanka I locate a steady, quiet – even grounded – part of myself.

In the jungle it's boiling hot, like the inside of a kiln – and this definitely helps with the stillness. I hang out near the lake, snug in a hammock's sling, tracking a gecko that slides across the ground, watching a bright tropical flower – its folds and buds and openings and the way it sways. I follow the splash of a shadow moving across the grass. I could stay there all day – and so I do. I have nowhere else to be. Days pass this way. I lose track of time. It's only hunger and a darkening sky that rouse me.

Those time-muddled and peaceful days in the garden in Sri Lanka remind me of a song Leonard Cohen wrote after many years in a Zen Buddhist monastery. It was about the floating dust motes you see when a ray of light comes through a window and how if you look closely enough they seem to dance and are a thing of beauty. That's what you see when you are very, very still – an individual dust mote. If you are still enough, the world opens up to you somehow. Everything seems epic and beautiful and miraculous.

Is this why people drop everything and move to a jungle or a monastery or a religious order? The intoxicating pleasure of finally observing life writ small? And how to harness this feeling and turn it on at will?

It's not hard to see that the enemy of this state of almost ecstatic stillness is the internet. Back at home the internet runs my life. I wouldn't have a job without it. But when I'm in Sri Lanka it becomes apparent that the pace of the online news cycle is killing some quiet corner in me. The web never stops – and as a consequence my brain never stops. Walk behind my desk and you'll see twenty-plus different tabs open on two browsers, plus a heap of Word docs. I constantly toggle between these, email and Twitter.

I get agitated if the internet is slow, and anxious if I'm offline. And that's just my computer. My phone is a whole other story. My head is bowed more than sixty times a day to this digital deity, checking and refreshing and tapping out little messages.

It's not just that the internet and our phones contain a multitude of ways to entertain us. It's that they are so effective at taking us away from ourselves. And if there's anywhere a lot of us don't want to be, it's with ourselves. A meditation teacher told me years later that we get addicted to our phones 'because we want to avoid feeling something. It's a resistance to and a rejection of life. The phone is our anaesthetiser. The outer world we live in is mainly out of our control. On social media we get agreement and approval constantly. It's a safer world.'

A revelation I have in Sri Lanka is that all I need to feel alive and good is to walk into long grass and lie down there – for a long time, doing nothing in particular – and just feel. Ulpotha is set up for discoveries of this kind. It's a world before and beyond technology – electricity, even. Without electricity you cut off the possibility of a whole range of night-time activities. These include reading, watching TV, surfing the net and talking on the phone (there is no mobile signal either). When it gets dark, it really gets dark. Gas lamps are strung from trees around the jungle and the looming forms of villagers each carrying their own lamp gives the place a vibe like a tropical Narnia.

I'm forced to spend time with other people at night, playing backgammon or cards, strumming guitar, singing, dancing, swimming and talking. It is enchanting and gives me a glimpse into a way of life, almost pre-modern, that follows the light and the seasons. Some nights we gather around the lake and sit in a large, open tent to talk then chant. The chanting is a loosely organised initiative designed to calm us before sleep. The retreat works its magic. Maybe it's the yoga, meditation, rest, stillness and treatments – or maybe it's simply nature. But I'm moving slowly but surely away from the belief entrenched since childhood that God could be found in a church. I'm finding evidence of this mysterious, animating, unseen force everywhere here; mostly I'm finding it in nature. I know that if I am serious about having serenity that lasts longer than a holiday, I will need to reassess my relationship with technology.

My blissed state lasts for as long as I'm on retreat – which, sadly, is only another few days. After a week in Sri Lanka, I fly back overnight to Sydney and go directly from the airport to work. I turn on my phone and computer, fire up the internet and ask my colleagues in the newsroom what big stories I have missed. No one can remember.

reel into 2012 feeling battered and sorry for myself. I've moved back to Melbourne for a job and then three months in, as I am leaving for Christmas break, my boss calls me into her office and says, 'Here's your Christmas bonus, you're fab!'

Actually, she doesn't. She tells me the position isn't working out or I'm not working out – one of the two – and that today will be my last day.

All my colleagues have left for the Christmas break already. I find an empty cardboard box and start clearing out my desk. The scene – fired just before Christmas – seems too cliched to be real, yet it's actually happening.

I begin the long, sweaty walk up the hill to the station with the box. It is too full and starting to break, and I have to carry it with my arm under the bottom, like it's a heavy child. I ring Patrick, who is now also living in Melbourne. He comes to get me and has to hide a grin when he sees my broken box full of novelty mouse-pads and my teary eyes. But that night in his brutalist Fitzroy bunker (concrete floors like an Eastern Bloc abattoir, stair rails so sharp they slice your hand like prosciutto) he also promises to do something for me, which everyone should do for their friends when they have lost their job: *lend them money*.

I move back to my writing studio in the Nicholas Building in the city, where I go each day and sit at my desk like I have a lot of work to do – except I don't. Instead I apply for jobs that I don't get interviews for (my CV is looking like a blood bath – bodies everywhere), and ride the lifts up and down, chatting to the elevator operators (later immortalised in a Courtney Barnett song) who, like journalists, have jobs under threat because of technological change, and host fun Friday night parties. We dance to music coming from tinny speakers, as the lights of the Arts Centre spire and Flinders Street Station provide a glittering vista that feels less like a promise of a bright future and more like a mirage.

Patrick encourages me to look at this unexpected break from work, this lacuna in my schedule, as a gift after a hectic ten years. I don't need to be online all the time now. There's nowhere to go, no place to be – it's a good re-entry point into the search for serenity. I need it more than ever now. I am feeling really down about my situation – and am quite stressed about money. I apply for Centrelink, and trying to live on $450 a fortnight is fraught. My social life disappears and so does my confidence. My friends are mostly well established in their careers and don't think twice when booking a restaurant that will cost $100 a head. They always offer to pay my share, but shame always accompanies my gratitude. They own their own houses in tony suburbs. I'm renting a room in a share house. I've been poor before, but this time feels more frightening. It lingers like a winter flu that you can't shake off.

The months pass. What if I never get back on my feet? Don't people always say it's much more difficult to get a job when you're already unemployed? Each week dozens of letters from an 'employment provider' arrive with various appointments in bold. I have to do an English-language test and a skills test and meet with various skills assessors in a distant suburb who will place me in work (any work, they say – legislation mandates that you can't be choosy). While I'm being processed through the awkward hybrid of a heavily bureaucratic, partly privatised job-seeking system – with its long wait times on the phone and queues on cheap office carpet and bombardment of appointment times and letters – I ask myself, *What can I control in my life?* The job thing I can't really control; I just have to keep looking, and the process will take its course. The thing I can try to control is my response to this situation. Can I take the blows and still be chill? That's the real test, isn't it?

I just need to bed down some techniques to help me get there. I decide to visit a monastery again (I am more mature now, not so easily spooked), to see if I can access serenity through routine, silence and prayer, and a silent meditation retreat, which draws on more Eastern traditions.

I book a few nights at an Anglican monastery in central Victoria. It has the same prayer schedule and emphasis on silence as New Norcia but, being Anglican, there's less separation between men and women. I'm allowed to eat with the monks and nuns. I can also talk at mealtimes. It's only after dinner that the monks descend into what they call the Great Silence, which lasts from 8pm until early-morning prayer the next day.

I'm prepared for the nightmares, the anxiety, the silence and the sometimes unexpected breakthroughs that can happen on retreat in a monastery. I know you have to be still, open yourself up and almost … wait, if you want to touch on any sort of mystical experience. Unlike in New Norcia, I'm the only guest here (which is *weird*) but, just like in New Norcia, my days are punctuated with prayer and silence. The spaces in between the prayer sessions are to be used for personal contemplation.

The guest building is semi-modern, built in the 1970s or '80s, and overlooks a large brown lake that's badly depleted after a long drought. There are crucifixes in every room and faded religious paintings, but otherwise everything – not just the lake – is brown: the carpet, the walls, the tiles. It feels like I'm the guest of an elderly relative with a strong religious bent.

I realise, with some shame, how tied to a certain aesthetic I am. How can one truly contemplate higher things amid such drab surroundings? Where are the dreaming spires? At least New Norcia looked epic and strange. Outside, the sun beats down hot and the winds stir the stagnant water of the lake. In the still heat of the night, mosquitoes buzz around the monastic single bed like a moving shroud, keeping my mind occupied with thoughts of pest control rather than the contemplation of higher things.

Must be silent, I tell myself. *Be Zen!* 'The quieter you become, the more you can hear,' says American spiritual teacher Ram Dass. Yet in my head I run a continuous commentary, like I am a whinger on TripAdvisor rating everything from the meals to the masses – and finding them lacking. I'm so used to judging everything, having an opinion on everything, running it through a filter that labels every experience 'good' or 'bad', that I'm unable to stop even when it's pointless to do so. What does it matter if I don't admire the decor? Who cares? But my mind, used to constant stimulation, locks on to anything it can find in an effort to stop from falling into uncomfortable silence. There is abundant stillness at this retreat centre yet my mind is labelling this stillness as boredom – and driving this furious inner monologue.

Outside prayer time, I'm left mostly to my own devices (literally – there is no tech ban here) and wander around the desiccated lake. It's unlike a retreat in, say, Bali, where every minute is timetabled and the spiritual experience is curated, with participants constantly kept entertained and engaged. But it's the quiet and emptiness that attract people here. The abbot tells me they come to the monastery for the chance to evaluate their lives.

Apart from the second morning, when I sleep in and miss the 4.30am prayer bell, I attend all the services dotted throughout the day. It's mostly just me and the monks and nuns, but every now and again a fresh face – a person from a nearby farm, perhaps – scurries in and takes a place in the pew. I let the singing and the prayers wash over me, and I pray for things for myself and others – things big and small. (*Oh please, Lord, let me be loved. Oh please, Lord, get me a job.*) And I wonder about all the monks, in all these quiet and lonely retreat centres around the world, and all the prayers each day, thrown up into the sky like paper planes.

The visitors who come to this monastery aren't necessarily spiritual seekers. 'A lot of people just come looking for a sense of space,' the abbot tells me. 'Sometimes they come from stressful situations. Some people go to a B&B or a pub but they don't have the same ambience and peacefulness.' A retreat, he says, is a chance to 'bring the warring voices within your heart to stillness. It's about creating peace within yourself. You have the power within yourself to make changes in how you think and react. Solitude can give people the opportunity to bring about change in their own life.'

I am not there yet. I cannot seem to dive in and have that necessary deep look at myself – at least not here. Instead I fret about money, making calculations on my phone about how much rent I can pay before my savings run out. My time in Sri Lanka, the beautiful stillness I found there, seems like something from a lifetime ago. Why can't I just drop into that state whenever I want? Is it like peak fitness, and once the goal has been reached it must be assiduously maintained?

When it's time to go, the abbot takes me back to the main street. It's an old country town with wide, tree-lined streets, pretty but also hot, dry and still. Apart from the flies, there's an air of life suspended. I browse the shops and buy a shirt I can't afford with beautiful stitching down the front, killing time until the bus comes to take me back to Melbourne. I see one of the monks in the dairy aisle of the supermarket, sweating in his heavy black robes, the rope of his belt swinging. He's like someone dropped into the present from medieval times, the light in the yoghurt section shining back towards his face. *The light in me bows to the light in you.*

**

The next retreat I attend is only a few days later, but it's quite different. It's a silent meditation retreat at a Buddhist centre on the outskirts of Melbourne. The meditation is mindfulness and the vibe is spiritual, not religious.

With its focus on meditation, I hope that this retreat will allow me to drop into stillness and access a serene core that I'm sure lies under layers of noise but have so far been unable to access in any meaningful way since Sri Lanka. I want to take my cues from the ocean: turbulent on the surface, but with still, unchanging depths below. And there's the hope, too, that by developing my inner serenity I will be better able to cope with blows such as losing my job, the vulnerability and uncertainty of being unemployed. Right now I'm not feeling grounded enough to take the knocks.

A number of books illustrate the concept of untapped internal wisdom and serenity with the proverb of the beggar. It goes something like this: a beggar has been sitting on a box for years, asking for money from passers-by. One day a dude stops and says, 'What's in the box?' The beggar says, 'I've been sitting on it for years but I have no idea.' Finally the beggar splits the box open and, amazingly, a treasure of gold bursts onto the ground. He's been sitting on it all this time and never even knew.

All humans are the beggar, and, according to spiritual teachers, it is through stillness we become aware of and break open the box of treasure we are sitting on. The treasure is serenity. We can't get to that place via our phones; we have to go inwards.

Thich Nhat Hanh, a Vietnamese Buddhist monk, writes: 'Everything inside and around us wants to reflect itself in us. We don't have to go anywhere to obtain the truth. We only need to be still and things will reveal themselves in the still water of our heart.'

Franz Kafka says: 'You do not need to leave your room. Remain sitting at your table and listen. Do not even listen, simply wait, be quiet, still and solitary. The world will freely offer itself to you to be unmasked, it has no choice, it will roll in ecstasy at your feet.'

'Stay put! For godsakes, stay still!' they all seem to be saying.

Imagine the world rolling in ecstasy at our feet, rather than the streams of data that roll off our screens then slip through our fingers, leaving no trace except agitation. While certain practices in the wellness industry are dubious (detox, meh), it's hard to argue with the quest to be more still, calm and contemplative. And here's the other thing – stillness costs you nothing. Yet it is the battle between stillness and distraction that we must fight anew every day. No one I know even acknowledges this battle exists.

**

Of the twenty of us attending the silent retreat in Healesville, some are fresh out of long-term relationships, others are dealing with stressful lives, family situations or businesses, and some people come on retreat every year, almost as a rebooting exercise.

The days start at 6am with meditation, followed by yoga, before participants gather for a vegan breakfast (incredibly delicious), which is eaten in silence. The setting in the Victorian bush is peaceful and quiet – there is a small woodland area (out walking one day, I see another participant literally hugging a tree) and below us, a really green valley – the sort you might see in a butter commercial – rolls out. One night I see a wombat walking slowly past my cabin, and during the day summer butterflies cluster above my head, moving cutely like GIFs.

I'd discovered Aruna, the meditation teacher, via another Google search, and by the end of my time with him, I appreciate the luck of that random result. Aruna says a lot of things that weekend that hit the mark. But before the talking, there is a lot of silence – crucial to helping people evaluate their lives. 'There is a busyness and craziness to most people's lives,' Aruna says, 'and if people were to stop and look inwards, the activity of the mind would also be seen as busy and crazy.'

After several days of silence and hours of meditation, people transform, Aruna tells me. 'The tension in their faces releases and they become more relaxed. Stress levels reduce. It's amazing to witness. It's like they are in a different place, like an old part of them has dropped away.'

People of all ages come to Aruna's retreats, held here and in India. Some come because they feel dissatisfied, or sense there is more potential to their lives and something is holding them back. 'There are always patterns from the past that are unresolved,' says Aruna. 'By turning inwards and by just "being" with these patterns, sooner or later a deeper insight dawns with a feeling of release. Then there is a resolution.'

Some participants are facing a big decision and the retreat creates a space so they can work it out. 'Sometimes it's not time to make a decision but the mind always wants to know. When a decision doesn't immediately happen, the mind impatiently worries. If there is trust and patience, the true answer will eventually arise from deep within with absolute certainty.'

This is the state I am trying to access – the place deep within, where knowledge forms with absolute certainty, the rich seam of inner wisdom that lies dormant. The gold box that I've been sitting on all this time.

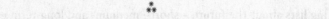

There are some experienced meditators on the retreat, as well as relative newbies like me. When it comes time to break the silence and ask questions, the beginners raise their hands and ask, 'How do I stop the thoughts from coming?' or 'What if my leg aches and I need to change positions?' The more experienced ones ask questions focused on sensations, rather than thoughts.

One guy in his twenties who doesn't wear shoes all weekend reports feeling a fire sensation in his chest and throat when he meditates. Another guy with long, silky brown hair reports seeing the colour purple.

I want fire and purple too. Instead I get an interesting mix of anxiety (worries and fears buzz in my head, louder than usual), personal insights and lengthening periods of feeling sort of blank. The blank feeling is good – it feels like I imagine the sensation of serenity might feel: clear, like water, an emptiness that's not particularly troubling, that doesn't feel like a lack.

Aruna talks about how we unconsciously process things. It usually goes something like this: action, reaction, contraction, tension. 'The reaction is where a lot of blockage comes from – so react differently,' he advises.

There are other lessons. One of the most important is to live in the present. 'You are here,' Aruna says several times a day, meaning, 'You are where you are meant to be.' This is a hard one for me. Am I really meant to be unemployed right now? How to feel comfortable in this uncomfortable place? Going on Centrelink is not part of my life plan. I'm a striver and so are all my friends. We are ambitious and push for what we want. Sometimes my life looks chaotic on the outside, but don't be fooled. I'm constantly writing lists about the future – short-, medium- and long-term goals; where I want to live; where I want to write; where I want to be; how to divide up the year. Always plotting and planning, I am, scribbling in my little journals.

But we are told to stay firmly in the present. The past is a graveyard. The future is not here yet; it doesn't exist.

This radical acceptance of wherever you are *right now* can be life-changing if you take it on board. It means resisting nothing, because whatever is happening to you is supposed to be happening. If you resist nothing then significant levels of unhappiness would disappear immediately. But resisting nothing is, of course, easier said than done. And it seems a bit passive to just accept the status quo. Where does ambition fit into this philosophy? And social change?

In the afternoon sessions there is a Q&A and I ask a lot of questions about this. (It's great to talk again!) Are social justice and this yogic way of life incompatible? After all, social change only happens when we resist and push back against conditions we find intolerable.

I go back and forth with this notion with Aruna, but don't get the answer that I want to hear – which is that sometimes you must push really hard against the grain of life to effect change, that resistance can cause suffering, but sometimes it's the best and only path to take. I mean, look at Gandhi...

After three days of fatigue, a low-level hum of anxiety, boredom and agitation, on day four I feel clear – that is, I feel nothing, or neutral. According to the other meditators, this is a good sign. Sitting still for hours on end is more comfortable than before and emptying my mind out becomes easier. I am just a blank, mass of cells sitting in a room. Time passes ... somehow. The past is a graveyard. The future doesn't exist. This is life lived in the eternal now. Thoughts come and go but don't stick around for very long. Is this serenity? I don't know. There haven't been any enormous revelations but there have been some modest insights. Some come as 'flashes' during meditation, others are just lurking around – stuff in the back of my brain that I haven't got around to sorting out yet. Some sound like banal platitudes (*Life is short! Be more vulnerable in your relationships! Appreciate your friends! Be grateful for your health!*), but when they come to me in the silence of meditation, it's like my heart is talking to me, not my head.

This is all good progress, and more than worth the price of admission, but I can't help but feel a little jealous of those who get the special effects – the fire and the visions and the chorus line of Hindu gods.

Meditation retreats can work – they allow you to dip out of your regular patterns for a bit and see your life as a stranger might see it. They're an evaluation vacation. After that first retreat with Aruna I'm hooked. The experience is a lot less confronting than going to New Norcia, and more immersive than the urban retreat I did in London. But life doesn't suddenly change or get better after one week away meditating. I return to Melbourne and my future is still uncertain, money tight, and I have a bunch of Centrelink and job centre appointments to attend. Samsara's a bitch, dude – or as Bowie would have it, we're always crashing the same car – and often, after the retreat, I find myself making the same mistakes or poor decisions time and time again. Aruna had said that 'there are always patterns from the past that are unresolved'. If you turn inwards and 'just be' with these patterns, eventually a resolution will come. But when? When do these resolutions occur? I want serenity now!

t's approaching the middle of the year and I still don't have a job – not a job-job, a proper job – not since I left that office with my broken box and fat tears. I'm teaching journalism at Monash University for around six hours a week, getting bits of freelance work and planning an escape to New York. I've found an apartment on the Upper West Side, a journalists' visa and some leads on work. I can't make it in Melbourne but I just might make it in New York. All that autumn I sing in the shower of my share house, 'If I can make it there, I can make it anywhere, except probably for Melbourne, yeah, yeah, yeah.'

In the months before I leave for America I go to Bikram yoga most days and spend the rest of my time in the writing studio at the Nicholas, marking essays. I'm poor and life is fairly quiet and boring.

So when a travel-writing opportunity comes up for a flying visit to a high-end, state-of-the-art wellness facility in the Philippines, I jump at it.

This place leads the world in raw food cuisine, but is even more popular for its *no food* cuisine, as evidenced by the number of people lying by the pool drinking juices and shakes in lieu of meals. The facility takes a scientific approach, testing and analysing your blood on the first day. They promise serenity via daily yoga and meditation sessions, as well as an amazing day spa.

Despite the deprivations that await, the Farm, a spa and integrated health resort (meaning there is a medical clinic onsite) is supposed to be out-of-this-world gorgeous. Villas, some with their own swimming pools, are placed at decent intervals on a huge, manicured estate. There are coconut groves, swimming pools, yoga pavilions, a restaurant and meditation huts. Peacocks wander past the sun lounges and there are approximately four staff per guest. Like so many luxurious health retreats, the spell only works if you don't think too much about where you are – if you pretend you don't have your own swimming pool and personal trainer in one of the poorest countries in the world.

Manila is a ninety-minute bus ride from the airport. On and on, as far as the eye can see, there is a muddy brown line of cardboard houses and people sleeping or sitting out the front on their makeshift stoops. I have never seen a slum before – and for that I need to thank the person pulling out the numbers in life's lottery. But now, in the taxi, I recognise it straightaway. It looks like all the pictures on the television news and in newspapers, the same visuals from Rio to Jo'burg to Haiti to Lagos: people in makeshift, temporary housing that is, of course, *not* temporary because it's not like anyone is going anywhere. The shelters are made of cardboard and look like they might at any moment slide into the muck (a river, a creek, a sewerage outlet?) that runs past their homes.

In Manila I stay with my friend Jackie, another former UN worker, now employed at one of the big Asian development banks. She and her friends Justin and Nat have just been to the crucifixions that happen outside Manila each Easter. They are *actual* crucifixions. We flick through photos on Justin's phone. There are real nails being driven through real hands. Justin's pants are flecked with blood from standing too close while a guy was getting nailed to the cross.

It's a visceral trip – Justin and Nat are also going to the Farm and the first thing they want to know is if I'm going to do a colonic. The place is famous for them. Euuughhh ... colonics! I shudder at the word, having a strong poo taboo. But colonics have a long history – they were performed in Egyptian times, with hollow reeds and river water. And in the time of Queen Victoria upper-class children received weekly colonics from a governess. Known as the 'Victorian enema', it sometimes coincided with weekly whippings and punishments, and the practice therefore left a sexual legacy on a generation of children. According to a sexual fetish forum I stumble across (one doesn't *visit* fetish forums, they are always *stumbled across*), 'So many boys and girls became sexually oriented to whipping and flagellation that it became known in Europe as the "English vice".'

During a colon cleanse, large amounts of water, sometimes with added extras such as herbs or coffee, are flushed through the colon using a tube inserted into the rectum. In some cases, smaller amounts of water are used and are left to sit in the colon before being removed.

This is another variation on the detox theme: our organs become worn-out over time, and need to be cleaned like a sewer system that is clogged from overuse. Old lumps of meat putrefy and become impacted on the internal wall of the colon. They stay there for years, rotting. This disgusting coating creates sluggish digestion and lack of blood flow, and contains parasites or pathogenic gut flora that cause poor health. This condition is known as autointoxication, and our large and small intestines need to be flushed out by throwing a heap of water through them.

But there is no science behind it. In 1919 a *Journal of the American Medical Association* paper debunked autointoxication, and according to Christopher Wanjek, author of the books *Bad Medicine* and *Food at Work*, 'Still to this day, direct observations of the colon through surgery and autopsy find no hardening of faecal matter along the intestinal walls.'

Yet colonics continue to be popular. In the late 1990s the *Journal of Clinical Gastroenterology* noted that colonics were making a comeback, publishing a paper entitled 'Colonic irrigation and the theory of autointoxication: a triumph of ignorance over science'.

In the wellness world, to be *clean* – to eat clean and to be clean on the inside – is next to, or even ahead of Godliness.

**

On Easter Saturday, the day I am due to go to the wellness facility, I wake up at 5am, somewhere in Manila's diplomatic district, beside a swimming pool and an empty bottle of champagne. It is still dark, warm and quiet. I am grateful that in my sleep I haven't rolled into the pool and drowned. The ambassador is away and his adult children had a party the night before. Yesterday at lunch – in a formal dining room at a long, long table where everyone was seated at least a metre apart – I consumed an entree of salami, two helpings of lamb, and, as the afternoon wore on, a lot of prosecco.

Later, waist-deep in the pool, drunker than I wanted to be, I was passed something strong that had been packed into a pipe. It felt like inhaling bitumen. It was a good Good Friday. Midnight ticked over. More cigarettes were sent for. A bottle of gin was opened. I stayed in the water for hours, turning into a warm prune. People came and went. We played Marco Polo and listened to Simon and Garfunkel. The night was close, like being in a comfortable old sock, and it felt okay to sleep outside, not even under a towel.

In a few hours a car is coming to take me to the spa, where I'll be staying for a week, consuming raw vegan food, doing yoga and maybe even trying a colonic in an attempt to cleanse myself. Serenity, something like the empty feeling I had on Aruna's retreat, will follow – I hope.

I roll away from the swimming pool, disgusted with myself. Here I am again, on this cycle that I despise but can't seem to escape – swinging between wellness and hedonism.

The Farm is lousy with staff, many walking around in lab coats. You can't move without a person offering you a refreshing chilled face towel, and every time a palm frond drops to the ground one of the worker guys in a bright jumpsuit springs onto the path and sweeps it away with a large broom.

Some of the guests take a 'wellness' package, which includes meals, an exercise regime with personal training, and spa treatments such as massage. All the food at the Farm is raw vegan – tiny portions of granola with nut milk, raw vegetables on skewers, cashew mousse – and, despite my initial hesitation, it's totally delicious, except for the corn cakes, which taste like dough and stick to the roof of your mouth.

But people mainly go there to detox, refraining from eating anything except for a few weird-looking shakes that are served at intervals throughout the day. The detoxers lie by the pool in the midday sun, glazed and still. It is oppressively humid, and sweat just courses from and off you like the plumbing in your body has gone badly awry. You don't just sweat in the Philippines, you leak. But sometimes a breeze passes across the grounds, rippling the surface of the swimming pool, stirring the pages of the fasters' magazines. The fasters are drowsy and don't even notice the pages turning. It's all a bit like a David Hockney painting.

Twice a day the people by the pool are escorted by a nurse down the long grove of palms for their colonics, their waste pumped from them through clear plastic tubing and deposited God knows where.

'I've lost inches from my waist,' one faster tells me in the clinic waiting room on my first day. She's nursing a heat pack against her abdomen and swallows a hefty pill to replace good bacteria in the colon after it has been flushed out. The whites of her eyes are brilliant, her frame gaunt. I wonder if she has cancer or if she has just been fasting for a long time. She tells me this is her thirteenth day in a row of colonics.

I see a doctor for an assessment soon after arriving. I have a hangover and my back has kinks in it from sleeping on the ground near the swimming pool. My blood is taken and analysed, and the results aren't good.

Have I by any chance been exposed to heavy metal? Second-hand smoke? Building sites?

I watch my cells drifting across the monitor.

'See that?' says the doctor. 'You have sputniks in your platelets.'

That, apparently, is not a good thing. I feel that emotion you never want to feel in a doctor's surgery: fear.

My profile, she tells me, is that of a 'lifelong meat eater'. A colonic is recommended as the first step in cleaning out my body.

'No way, Jose,' I tell her.

In the restaurant Justin and Nat debate whether or not to have a colonic. Nat has always been curious. 'Princess Diana used to have them,' he says. He's seen a nurse at the Farm who explained the two types of procedures: the colonic, which works on the lower intestine and involves coffee being pumped into your butt, and the colema, which is more intense, and cleanses both the upper and lower intestines with a 'machine'.

'I think I'm going to have a treatment,' says Nat, using the term we have all decided is more palatable than saying the word 'colonic' out loud. 'May as well while I'm here.'

'I'll have a treatment if you have one,' Justin says to me.

'I don't think I'll have one.'

The next day we meet again.

'Have you had your treatment?' I ask Nat anxiously.

'Yes, it was fine. I feel much lighter.'

Nat is skipping lunch as he is having another treatment in the afternoon. He looks serene, not at all disturbed or freaked out.

'Your eyes look clearer,' Justin says to Nat. We look into Nat's eyes, bright and white – not cloudy like mine usually are.

'Mmm, I suppose they are,' says Nat, almost absently. He is spacing out before our eyes.

'You're turning into that luminous, gaunt, fasting woman,' I tell him.

Over the next few days, he reports that his waste has taken on the texture and colour of what he has just eaten: 'Orange poos after eating those carrots for lunch,' he says, and we hang on every word – fascinated and grossed out.

While holding out on having a treatment, I do other things at the Farm that make me feel, at least superficially, very serene. I eat only vegan, raw food, go to bed at 8pm and wake refreshed without an alarm at 6am. I swim in the waterfall pool, go on a morning power walk with the Farm's personal trainer, do yoga in an outdoor pavilion and loll on a sun lounge by the pool. I have an 'under the stars' massage, a 290-minute epic that takes place outside – under the stars – and involves being coated in a chocolate scrub, then soaking in a tub of warm coconut milk, then having a Filipino massage.

But still the spectre of the *treatment* hangs over my stay.

Using the toilet in private is how I have generally done it all my life. The door is always *shut*. The exception being, of course, before I was toilet trained and had to be coaxed and cleaned by a parent.

And so it is again at the Farm when I finally relent (I am worried about my negative blood work). Grace is 'doing me', and staff promise me she is very experienced as they lead me down the path to where she is waiting, smiling, reassuring in her starched white uniform. She stands outside the door of the Colonics Room. It is immaculately clean. I don't know what I was expecting – a charnel-house? Excrement on the walls? But it is sparkling and, even more surprising, odourless.

'I've never done this before and I'm kind of scared,' I tell Grace. She says all the right things and is very soothing. I get changed into a hospital gown and she tells me to lie on my back and then slide down this bench thing and raise my knees. By this stage I am perspiring and my breathing is uneven. I'm not just 'kind of scared' – I'm terrified. I am not sure why this procedure scares me so much. Is it having a stranger *there*? The thought of my bowel perforating and being reliant on a colostomy bag for the rest of my life? Or the horror at seeing my shit being pumped out of me?

'Keep breathing,' Grace tells me. The urge to hold her hand is strong.

Here's what happens. You lie on a long bench with your legs either side of a sort of potty-shaped hole with a bowl underneath it. The nurse gloves up and sticks a lubed finger, then a tube, up your bum, then runs coffee through your lower intestines via the tube. The muck, as well as the coffee, ends up in the bowl. The nurse massages your stomach while the water filters through and you push it out. Maybe it's because I'm whimpering slightly and the nurse is so soothing, but I really do feel like a helpless baby.

I find the treatment more bearable if she keeps me distracted. I conduct what is effectively a potty-side interview to keep her talking. 'What sorts of people do this? Can you do this if you have colon cancer? How many times should one have this procedure?' She says people who have regular colonics are mainly business people who travel a lot for work and their internal systems are disrupted by all the different time zones. It's recommended as a preventative measure for colon cancer but they don't recommend it for people with colon cancer, and 'you should have this once a year' as a sort of maintenance exercise.

The treatment is in no way painful but the idea of it breaches some pretty entrenched psychological barriers. There are big

taboos about shitting in front of other people – even in the med-
icalised, white-coat, highly hygienic setting of a health farm. It's
impossible just to discard decades of private privyings. Yet here I
am – in thirty (strange) minutes I have crossed the Rubicon.

Back in reception I nurse a heat pack against my stomach and
take a big pill meant to replace lost gut flora.

Colonic irrigation can disrupt the gut's natural flora, and
flooding the colon with water can lead to loss of electrolytes and
other balancing agents in the body. If done roughly or not under
supervision, there is a risk the bowel could tear. Of course the
Farm is anything but rough, and I suffer no ill effects. But, apart
from feeling 'emptier', it doesn't seem to do much. That said, I
don't suffer from gut issues or any of the digestion problems that
drive people to the procedure in the first place. So I cross colonic
irrigation off my wellness bucket list and never really think about
it again. I am certainly not making it part of any health regime
back home.

The interesting thing is not so much the colonics themselves – which are gross – but why they have found a place in the
modern wellness industry. One colonic irrigator interviewed by
the Straight Dope website explains, 'You can watch everything
come out and see what you're really made of or what you've been
holding on to for days, months, or years! You can let go into a completely enclosed system – no smell – no mess.'

The market for colonics – particularly in upmarket health
spas – is as much driven by deeper psychological needs as health
concerns. You lie down, breathe, and just ... *let go*. It all comes
out – the things that were making you stuck, the things that were
making you sick, the things you were holding on to for years and

years and years. You watch the toxic stuff that was stuck inside you disappear down the tube. It's gone forever. The feeling of lightness descends.

Could this be the key to serenity? Could it be as simple as releasing your shit? Let it go, let it go …

If only it were really so easy.

After three months in New York I am close to making it. Almost, almost, almost. I'm down to the final round for a job with a global human rights campaign group. I'm all about Syria and injury compensation for illegal Mexican workers on the construction sites of Texas, and worker safety in factories in China. At night I prep by reading about all the troubles in the world and drafting possible solutions. In my ground-floor apartment in Park Slope, I'm a one-woman UN. You got a human rights problem, yo, I'll solve it. The interviews – I've done around eight so far – are weird, more like intense, non-sexual dates where I'll meet members of the organisation in semi-social situations and we'll talk about all the troubles in the world, and – OMG, where did you get those great shoes?!

In the meantime, as the selection process rolls on, I accept an assignment to do some travel stories in Indonesia for a newspaper.

The trip is a deep dive into the world of luxury hotels, villas, butlers and swimming pools. The wellness industry is booming – particularly in Bali, where the spiritual-industrial complex keeps a large segment of the tourist and long-term visitor market ticking over. Zoom in closer on Google Maps, and there's Ubud – wellness ground zero. It has everything you could want, from the traditional healers to the upmarket yoga classes, all of it cheap as chips for Westerners. And so we go and binge on it. Which is what I planned to do, too.

When I land, it's minutes to midnight and a young Balinese guy called Mus collects me from the airport. We bounce along the back roads, our way illuminated by torchlight and a slow-moving procession. There is a giant papier-mâché bull on the tray of the ute in front of us and Mus says there's a body inside the bull. They are bound for a cremation ceremony.

It's my first trip to Bali and I feel like I am decades late to the party. Bali was a place you avoided if you had any sense. It was somewhere you flew over on the way to Europe. Bogans went there for cheap beer and T-shirts. The streets were full of drunk Aussies with braided hair, tattoos and sunburn. That's what I thought, anyway, before I found myself on this road, inhaling what I now recognise as the quintessentially Balinese smell: jasmine, frangipani, sewage and rotting garbage. I've only just landed and already the place is blowing my mind. It seems mysterious, complex and unknowable in a similar way to India. Australia by comparison feels two-dimensional, washed out with too-bright sun, box-like and functional – a Howard Arkley painting to Bali's Paul Gauguin.

Mus wears frangipani flowers tucked behind his ears, blasts Justin Bieber and asks what I do. On hearing that I'm a journalist bound for Ubud, he says, 'Just like Liz Gilbert in *Eat, Pray, Love*.' I bridle at this. No – I'm not looking for love in Bali. But I suppose that, like Gilbert, I am looking for serenity and balance. It was – unsurprisingly – hard to find in New York.

After only a few days I realise it's impossible to have a wholly material experience in Ubud. The spiritual is everywhere – not just in the remarkable ceremonies that fill the streets, weaving around and sometimes absorbing the tourists, but also in the religion itself. Around 90 per cent of Balinese are Hindu with a unique strain of animism, despite the predominantly Islamic population of mainland Indonesia. In Ubud and the surrounding villages, there are temples on every corner – sometimes tiny, family ones, others open to the public, so open that you can join a ceremony and for a brief time be folded into the religion. From the women making delicate offerings to appease the spirits each morning to the ravens for sale in the marketplace for evil spells – the inhabitants of Ubud have one foot in this world and the other foot in another.

The tourists I meet here are also of the spiritual-seeker variety. I overhear two Australian women at an organic cafe in Ubud: 'Have you done breath work? Oh my God, you fall down on your knees, you scream, you shake, you laugh, like that thing in Adelaide – you know that thing? Well, they do it here.'

The woman next to me has barely drawn breath. 'I'm getting a colonic tomorrow. The only ones I could get into are on Thursday and Monday. Dry skin brushing – who does that? My name is down for the Tantra workshop.'

I'm drinking a delicious juice of orange, carrot, papaya and basil, wanting the woman to stop talking, wanting her to keep going. I'm meeting lots of people like her in Bali – working on the great project of self, gathering in the health food shops and vegan cafes that are everywhere here, gorging themselves on cheap therapies.

Wellness in the West doesn't come so cheap. Back in Sydney you have to be a millionaire to practise wellness to the full. But here in Bali you can have this millionaire's wellness lifestyle – the organic food, the juices, the yoga, the meditation classes and the therapies – at a fraction of the cost. So the part-time models and yoga teachers and student naturopaths flock here. This cohort, clutching a turmeric juice as if it were the elixir of life, are easy to mock, and tender prey to those offering a variety of New Age treatments that are at best a waste of time and at worst cause harm. But hadn't I gone to see a palm reader up a rickety staircase in Covent Garden? And hadn't I seen the elderly tarot card reader who operated from a park in Yangon? Did I not, on some level, *believe*?

After a few days eavesdropping in juice bars, I decide to become more open to the spiritual side of Bali. When in Rome, and all that ... Anyway, Ubud's tourism-creating spiritual-industrial complex is where the real and vivid energy in the town can be found. It's not the scant nightlife (everything seems to shut down around 10pm), or the terrifying monkeys that hiss then relieve you of your iPhone on Monkey Forest Road. The main game here is the spiritual one. It's word of mouth and secret doorways, a kind of all-you-can-eat buffet for seekers.

The main religion in Ubud for white people is yoga. And the place where they come to worship is the massive Yoga Barn, with its cathedral-in-the-tropics ceilings, polished floors and open-air cafe. It runs classes from dawn until dark, seven days a week, with instruction in English, offering everything from hatha to 'sound healing' workshops. The crowd is the global yoga set, a mixture of tourists and expats with tattooed, toned bodies, who you might also see at retreats in Mexico, Goa or Costa Rica. The teachers hail from around the world, but in my week there I am taught mostly by American instructors.

We are packed in rows, with a soothing view of green palms and a pond just beyond the glass-panelled walls that can be opened to let in a cooling breeze. All around us are rice paddies and jungle.

In the first class I take, yin yoga, we are given tennis balls to put under our hips and thighs to roll on. We are encouraged to talk, which I find to be a great distracter from my pain.

'Why does it hurt so much?' I bellow from the back.

'Who asked that?' says the vaguely intimidating, heavily tattooed instructor.

'Me!'

'Fascia and tissue. Trauma, particularly fear, is stored in the legs. Remember when you were young and just learning to walk? And your parents were saying, "Be careful!" Well, you can store that fear in your legs.'

Around me, grown men are groaning as if they are giving birth. I am finding rolling around on a tennis ball close to unbearable. I must be storing a lot of trauma. I wonder if this is why people come to Ubud for a holiday and stay for years – they discover pain they didn't even know they had, and the quest to fix it isn't quick.

The next day I try a different yin class (the slow, gentle yoga that I favoured so much before I did the vinyasa-heavy Modern Yogi project), this time at a place called Radiantly Alive. The vibe is mellow. A sign says, 'For karma points put your shoes on the rack.' Everyone here seems to know each other, and there is a lot of kissing and cries of 'Oh my God, haven't seen you since Seminyak!'

At the end of the class the instructors invite us all out to a bar that night to see some African drummers. There is a slipstream here, one that would be easy to fall into: Bali Buddha for a juice, then cross the road to Radiantly Alive for yoga, then African drumming … repeat. If you want to stay, like, *forever* you go to a place behind a juice shop and up some rusting stairs to a room where a Swedish woman who keeps envelopes fat with rupiah and US dollars on a card table, also cluttered with paperwork and passports.

I find a room for twenty-seven dollars a night above a Sufi meditation centre. Gloria, her white hair pinned up with frangipani flowers, is my host and meditation guide. Before moving to Bali she'd been a psychotherapist in Austria for more than thirty years. We pass pleasant morning hours drinking coffee in the garden, talking about the world and its problems.

I pump her for information. Is there one universal problem or theme that keeps cropping up? Is there one mistake we're all making over and over again? Gloria reckons the root of many people's problems is that they are not bold enough: they fall in love with someone but cannot tell them, they want to quit their job but they're too scared, they wish to leave their marriage but are frightened about being alone. If only we were brave, we might suffer less.

Some who do leave their husbands or are searching for some sort of better life end up in Bali. The place is lousy with divorcées. They pass through the guesthouse on their way to enlightenment, asking for directions to the *Eat, Pray, Love* healer Ketut's house or seeking the recommendation of decent healers or psychics.

'I think that stupid book ruined Bali for me,' says Gloria, being uncharacteristically negative. 'Women come to Ubud looking for a handsome Brazilian and they get a small Balinese and they are not happy.'

I'm not expecting romance. The vibe is off. In a place where everyone is working on themselves, the energy is curiously sexless. It's all focused inward.

*
**

Seeking serenity, I attend three meditation sessions guided by Gloria. The Sufi meditation we do as a group on the roof of her building, under the stars, is my favourite. It's like a mixture of prayer and dance, designed to rouse the soul and spirit and drop attachments to materialism. There are nine of us high above the treetops – all women, all wearing white, spinning and whirling to trance-like music with an accordion and a steady drumbeat that invokes some faraway souk.

Gloria tells me that movement meditations, not Vipassana (sitting meditation), are most suitable for the uninitiated. 'They are more appropriate for Western people, who have a hard time calming their minds. By doing action, the mind becomes focused on that – the breathing and the movement calms the mind and gives it a glimpse of peace.'

I tell her about my patchy, undisciplined history with meditation, the difficulty I have diving right down and staying there, my love of technology, my appetite for distraction. 'Meditation is essential for sanity,' she says. 'I am convinced no therapy works without meditation. You can go to a psychiatrist for twenty years but only meditation will heal neurosis.' And only meditation will get you to a place of serenity. She also believes that 'every psychic problem not resolved will usually show up in your body as an illness. Usually it's way later.'

Errr ... okay. I like the talk about meditation, but not this. The leap is too big, and anyway, there's no science there. Yet it's a dark belief held by many people I know – even the most sensible and secular of my friends. They'll hear of someone getting cancer and they'll nod and say, 'Well, yes, she was always stressed.'

**

An Australian businessman who runs a luxury hotel in Uluwatu in the south of Bali tells me he employs the services of healers for everything from stopping the rain at weddings to finding a lost master key. Another, very sensible, Englishman I speak to is convinced a healer has put a bad spell on his iPhone. A woman I meet who had a long-term stomach complaint says she was cured when a healer poked her in the foot with a stick. Then there is healing of the emotional kind.

People I meet in Ubud talk of a visit to the healer being an emotionally cathartic experience. The healers, they say, have the unnerving ability to stare deep into your heart and pull out your most submerged desires ... sometimes. A Bostonian I meet tells me she had lined up for hours to see a healer who was recommended highly on TripAdvisor. When they finally came eyeball to eyeball he told her, 'You have a big secret you are keeping.' She looks pissed off as she tells me, 'I've done a lot of work on myself. I don't have any secrets.'

Gloria recommends a healer but the experience apparently involves being 'shaken' for two hours a day in order to completely reconfigure my cells, so I pass and instead opt for someone more conventional. Riki is recommended by a friend of a friend. We meet in the tropical garden of a nearby hotel, and when he arrives he is wearing an enormous black motorbike helmet with the visor up. We walk to a daybed at the bottom of the garden and sit on it awkwardly, and he takes off his helmet.

'So, this healing lark, not really sure about it, but hi-ho let's go and all of that ...' I mutter.

Riki asks me to draw a number of objects on a piece of paper (a snake, a house, a fence, a door), which he then interprets, not very convincingly. Then he gives me some life advice, some of which is good, such as not to read the comments at the bottom of my articles. He follows this with a palm reading that sounds like an optimistic early-morning traffic report: all clear on the road ahead, a smooth journey awaits. Then he waves his arms in front of my body and, after a few minutes, looks very sad and says he really can't help me too much because I have too much doubt in the process.

I exhale, somewhat relieved, and settle into just talking to Riki. He tells me he's just making a name for himself, but has a knack for intuition, particularly with foreign women. He offers to throw in a chakra reading. We are losing light in the garden; the session has gone for two hours. I'm bored. It has been like a pantomime he's put on for an audience of one. Not a word of it feels true.

Riki asks me to close my eyes and lie down on the daybed. He looms above me – I can smell tea and cigarettes on his breath. I sense his hand, or at least the heat of it, travelling around my body. Once I sit up he tells me quite matter-of-factly, 'Your head is good, your heart is so-so, but you need to energise your sex chakra.' He offers to have sex with me to unblock it. 'It will make you clear,' he says clinically. With that, he stands up, puts on his helmet, gives me a hug and tells me to call him to arrange a time for the 'treatment'. The cost is around twenty dollars.

I am outraged and bewildered. It's *Eat, Pray, Love* through the mirror darkly. I stand in his hug like a lump, my heart racing, and after he leaves, I keep turning around in the garden as if there might be someone else there. But I'm alone. In the distance is the foreboding sound of a gamelan, an instrument I can seemingly hear constantly and am beginning to hate. I don't know what rankles the most – Riki's assessment that I am sexually frustrated, that my heart is 'so-so', the blatant sexual harassment, the grim thought of having sex with him, or the suggestion that *I* would have to pay *him*.

∗∗

I've chosen a retreat in Ubud. Doing it with me are sixteen other women ranging in age from their early twenties to their sixties. They have come from offices and deadlines, from personal crises or uncertain health. They have caught a Melbourne, Tokyo or Moscow red-eye and thrown their yoga mats in the overhead lockers. In the yoga pavilion where we sit in a circle and introduce ourselves, there is an air of nervousness but also of fatigue.

Having stayed before in retreat centres where the carpet is stained and the curtains traumatised, where the beds are a punishment and the food a form of self-flagellation, this venue is like a palace. There are Toblerones and Bintang beer in the bar fridge and two swimming pools with beanbags and daybeds. Our hosts are urbane and generous – and in a way are models of the good life. We do a lot of meditation and yoga but wine is brought out at dinner, and we are invited to a cocktail party at the nearby royal palace with weak martinis and golden sparkling wine. Bali is meant to be all about balance – and so it is here.

But, I wonder, how on earth do you *integrate* all this stuff when you're in the day-to-day trenches of adult existence? Is it even possible? It's a question I come back to time and time again – my samsara.

On the second night of the retreat we are given a white sarong and a white shirt with long sleeves. We put on these garments and are driven to a nearby temple for a purification ceremony. In single file we sink into the waist-deep water, our white robes floating up, twisting and dragging like sheets in a spin cycle. We then line up and move between ten fountains, ducking down and fully immersing our heads at every one. Each time we go under we must make a wish or let something go. Balinese come here for fertility rituals but also for purification. If something bad has happened to them or their family, this is the place to let it go.

Afterwards, my fellow retreat ladies and I sit in an area covered in grey headstones. It's getting on towards midnight. We make an offering at a shrine, and sit next to a group of Balinese who are singing low and quiet in tones that to my ears sound like the hymnal melodies of Christian missionaries. A priest moves along our row, scattering holy water on us, and presenting us with rice. Cats without tails move over the grey stones and the almost-full moon is as bright as a lamp, the air hazy with the smoke of incense, flowers crushed all over the ground. This and the singing, the darkness and the incredible stillness give the night some sort of ancient cast. I have to remember to breathe.

At some time, maybe around 1am, we go back to the car park. A TV is bolted to a pole and blasting some Indonesian soap opera; groups are still coming in to bathe, children in their parents' arms. We have some tea and eat some sweets and take the vans back to the retreat, our soaked clothes in bags at our feet.

I feel uneasy about the ceremony. Sure, the ritual is beautiful, and the aesthetics of the entire evening – the white gowns and the full moon and the graveyard – feel like a Bill Henson photograph. But ritual without religion? That seems strange, like it's been unclipped from history and the things that gave it meaning, and now it's just there, a free-floating form without substance – like a plastic bag. Are we in the West so bereft of our own traditions, and so arrogant about the traditions of others, that we think we can just put on a white robe, visit a temple and siphon some of the healing powers from someone else's god?

Yet by the end of the week, something strange has happened that leaves no room for cynicism or even rational thought. It's one of those rare moments, a consciousness-blowing experience that you only have once or twice in your life – if you are lucky! – and is utterly indelible.

On the last day, when everyone is tanned and floppy with a complete lack of stress and worry (so different from how they were that first night), we sit in the yoga pavilion and are told to write down the things we want to let go of. Each woman gets up, one by one, and throws her paper into the fire.

It's an old, familiar ritual, but by the time the second person has burnt their paper I am sobbing. I am also embarrassed. No one else is crying. Why the hell am I crying? The sobs move through me like a current, and strangely, despite the racket I'm making, I feel not sad or upset but deeply connected to not only the people in this circle but everyone on the planet. I've never felt like this before. I feel a profound sense of empathy and compassion for everyone, and I'm feeling it so much that the only commensurate physical response is these full, body-racking sobs.

With a mixture of awe and shame I guess that I am having what's called a religious experience, or some sort of spiritual awakening, which I try to hang on to because it feels so good. Better than anything I've ever felt. As soon as I try, it goes. The whole thing lasts maybe two or three seconds and feels like a flood.

We walk down to a river, where there is a Balinese dude singing and the yoga instructor mixing the ashes of all our combined fears and stuff we want to let go. He throws the ash in the river, which is flowing fast. I feel a shiver of disapproval because it's bad for the environment, but quash it because the action contains an allusion to something bigger – that this will be all of us one day, ashes in a bowl, returned to nature.

Later on I try to explain the sensations I felt at that moment to people – but really, there are no words. Also, it sounds very similar to a drug experience, which can be really boring to hear about if you weren't there. I try to capture the experience again with more retreats and meditation, and a lot of yoga – even ecstatic dancing – but it never makes a return visit.

I also know in ways I cannot articulate that the experience is truthful, that there is a divine, even if it's only to be found in nature or each other, rather than some omnipotent being. It's there.

I return to New York to an email saying I was unsuccessful for the campaigning job. From all the interviews and the quasi-social situations, they intuited that I was 'not a team player' and 'too independent'. I don't feel too disappointed, or at least not as disappointed as I once would have been. There's been a shift. I'm not knocked off balance so much. I'm filled with a feeling of inner calm, peace and serenity, and at the moment these qualities seem as essential as water and air. This time I want the feeling to last.

What I discover is that if you want to get serious about serenity, then you *need* a daily meditation practice. There are loads of different types – mindfulness, Vipassana, Zen, Kundalini and Vedic, just to name a few. I'd meditated with some excellent teachers such as Maitreyabandhu and Aruna, tried mindfulness and Zen, and all sorts of apps on my phone that tailor meditation for various circumstances: trouble getting to sleep, anger, heartbreak, long commutes.

But the premium, celeb-endorsed meditation is Transcendental Meditation – or TM, as its followers call it. Celebrity devotees include Katy Perry, Hugh Jackman and Madonna. I interview Heather Graham and she raves about it. 'TM calms you down. It helps you find that peaceful place inside yourself – so whenever your life is going a bit crazy, it reminds you how to be really centred,' she tells NBC. Jerry Seinfeld describes his twice-daily meditation practice as like 'a phone charger for your mind'. Russell Brand credits TM with helping him stay sober. Film director David Lynch, the sort of de facto father of this wave of celebrity TM, says the practice gave him 'effortless access to unlimited reserves of energy, creativity, and happiness deep within'. He's taken the technique to schools and prisons, and funds scientific studies into the benefits of meditation.

Early studies – not just Lynch's – have shown that it can increase immune function, lower blood pressure, decrease pain and inflammation at a cellular level, improve focus, attention and your ability to regulate emotion, and increase your level of compassion.

Although TM has been around for roughly 5000 years, it didn't come to mainstream Western attention until the Beatles went to India, learnt the technique from Maharishi Mahesh Yogi, had their minds blown and wrote the *White Album*.

Hollywood followed, then the business community. Yep – meditation can make you money! Ray Dalio, founder of Bridgewater, the world's largest hedge fund, told Reuters, 'I think meditation has been the single biggest reason for whatever success I've had.' It's no wonder some of the biggest global companies are introducing meditation in the workplace. Bloomberg ran a story headlined, 'To Make a Killing on Wall Street, Start Meditating', and executive coach David Brendel wrote in the *Harvard Business Review*, 'Mindfulness is close to taking on cult status in the business world.'

In 2015 the *New Yorker* examined the cross-pollination of corporate America and meditation: 'Meditation, like yoga before it, has been fully assimilated into corporate America. Aetna, General Mills and Goldman Sachs all offer their employees free in-office meditation training.'

The titans of the tech world are also enthusiastic meditators. The late Steve Jobs was an early adopter. And one of the Silicon Valley success stories is Headspace – a mindfulness app that has brought meditation to the masses. Downloads of the app had reached 5 million in 150 countries by 2016, according to the *LA Times*.

My colleague Mustafa, who I work with in a Melbourne newsroom, meditates before we start our shifts at 6am. This means he has to get up at 4am. He never complains about the early starts and always comes into work looking as fresh as a daisy (so fresh that he works part-time as a male model). The early starts and meditation seem to give him more energy, not less. He encourages me to give it a go.

But once I locate some TM teachers my jaw hits the floor. It's around $1500 to learn the technique. I don't have that type of cash right now.

A few months later I change jobs and cities – again. I love my new job – features editor at *Guardian Australia*, back in Sydney. But it's a broad remit and I feel overwhelmed almost immediately.

I start on Monday and two days later I have tightness in my chest. By Friday I'm in the doctor's surgery hooked up to a cardiogram, certain I'm about to have a heart attack. Nothing shows up. The doctor suggests that perhaps I was having an anxiety attack. I leave the surgery shaken. I need desperately to chill out. In other words my stress is causing me stress. I start looking for a meditation teacher in Sydney immediately.

Vedic is a similar technique to TM, but teacher Matt Ringrose charges $750, instead of thousands. It's still a lot of money but includes a week of tuition and an open door to his house every Monday night for group meditation. Every Monday night for the rest of my life, if I want it.

I attend an information session to see if it's for me. Matt teaches meditation from his home in Bondi, just a short walk from where I live. Upstairs, the meditation room is like an interiors catalogue – couches in pastel colours, some on-trend soft furnishings and then the balcony, which faces the sea.

At the information session there are four of us, including a woman so stressed and busy that she needs her PA to schedule toilet breaks in her diary. Her eyes are focused on the middle distance, she talks staccato and her foot whirrs with agitation. I have lived in a lot of cities, but this is yet another reminder of how, beneath the sun and the fun, Sydney is one of the most stressed of them all. At the end of the session, I sign up to learn Vedic meditation and, after raiding my savings, the next week I'm doing the course.

The first night is one on one. You have to bring an odd assortment of things – a white linen handkerchief, a fresh bunch of flowers and three pieces of sweet fruit. All are easy to come by except for the handkerchief, which no one seems to sell any more because it's not 1981. After I present the offerings I get my mantra – which I am told to keep secret – and then, without much further ado, we are meditating.

After the first meditation a very subtle but undeniable feeling comes over me – I feel slightly buzzed, grinning and happy. Maybe the meditation has released some sort of endorphins. It's not unlike the feeling after a really good workout. Each meditation I do with Matt that week is subtly different. Sometimes all goes smoothly and I achieve that elusive 'blank' feeling that I had a taste of when meditating with Aruna; sometimes I get bored, and time crawls; other times my mind is agitated and racing. The trick is just to repeat the mantra – a sort of mental white noise – and dispassionately observe what's coming up. Matt says the agitated and noisy meditations are nothing to be alarmed about: 'It's just the brain processing stress. It's all part of the process.'

After a week of meditating I feel a definite effect. My sleep becomes deep and unbroken – the sort of sleep that, when you come out of it, feels like you're surfacing from an anaesthetic. I would then groggily haul myself into a seated position (on my bed, covers off, back against the wall) for twenty minutes' meditation. During the week of the course, the anxious feelings immediately stop and my concentration improves. I don't feel as overwhelmed by my new job or the email load that has gone from around a dozen a day to more than a hundred a day.

The only issue is getting up early enough to meditate (although Matt reckons twenty minutes of meditation is worth several hours' sleep) – and finding somewhere to meditate in the afternoons.

It's not always practical to meditate in the mid-afternoon – as I find out when I walk around Flemington Racecourse, stepping over drunk people on Melbourne Cup Day, trying to find somewhere quiet to meditate. Every day I think I'm too busy to meditate twice a day, but Matt says that if you think you are too busy to meditate, then you need to meditate.

So I keep going, doing it twice a day, because I quite like it. My brain starts to crave these regular mini-breaks. As one meditator puts it in *GQ*: it 'taps an inner calm we all have, a calm that gives the brain a chance to settle and repair its frazzled neurons'.

My boss is sceptical: 'My father did TM – I don't think it works. You'll give it up soon enough. You're always doing these things then after one month dropping them. You have to do forty minutes a day, don't you? That's a lot of sitting. What's your mantra anyway?'

'I can't tell you,' I say, vaguely shocked she would ask. One of the things that's drummed into us in the course is that our mantra must be a secret.

'I bet there's one mantra,' says my boss. 'And they tell you to keep it a secret so that you don't find out that there's just one that they give out to everyone.'

'It's vacuum,' I say. 'Vacuum, vacuum, vacuum.'

'No, it's not.'

**

If the wellness industry were to be depicted in a food pyramid form, it's meditation that is the base that holds everything up. Which makes sense, doesn't it? There's no point rocking a hot body and having a clean liver and being able to backbend like a sabre if you are unable to control or at least *deal* with the blows, the bad moods, the existential angst, the disappointments and just general all-round sadness that is sure to come your way. Of course, meditation doesn't promise to rid you of these things, but what it does do is give you mental space – and perhaps the ability to hold the line as the waves crash over you.

Of all the wellness things I have tried for this book, it is meditation that there is the most love for. Adam Whiting, my Bondi yoga teacher, kept telling the class that even if we could not make a yoga class, we had to keep meditating. It also – for me – finally sticks. Matt has taught me how to integrate the Vedic method into my everyday life. There are no excuses. Finally, I become a meditator.

E ven though I didn't get that human rights campaigning job I went for in New York, I am working on my own projects. One thing I have been working on for a few years is a clemency campaign for two Australians on death row in Bali – Andrew Chan and Myuran Sukumaran. A few other death-penalty activists and I have been plugging away at a website and petition in a fairly low-key way for a while. The two men have been on death row for almost ten years, and the Indonesian government don't seem to be in any hurry to start executing prisoners.

Then in December of 2014 I am at work at the *Guardian* office in Sydney when an alert flashes on the wire service.

During a public lecture the newly elected Indonesian president Joko 'Jokowi' Widodo has emphasised that his government would not be merciful in dealing with narcotics-related crime. He advised he would reject requests for clemency for sixty-four drug traffickers currently on death row.

Things in life move fast and slow, and so it is with this. Over the next four months, our small campaign explodes into a world-wide movement.

In those early days of 2015 we are locked in a furious cycle of hope, despair, anxiety, sleeplessness, elation, depression and fear. On it goes. The men are transferred to the Nusa Kambangan prison – and execution site. Will the seventy-two-hour notice period be triggered now? Or is Jokowi playing chicken? There are vigils and press conferences and public pleas. Artist Ben Quilty organises the Music for Mercy concert, and more appeals are filed. We gather 250,000 signatures on the Mercy Campaign petition to stop the executions. But nothing – the petition, the exhaustion of all legal and diplomatic avenues, the appeals of various high-profile religious and political leaders – makes one jot of difference. At midnight on Tuesday 28 April Andrew and Myuran are killed by firing squad.

Andrew is buried in south-west Sydney on Friday.

Myuran just down the road on Saturday.

On Monday I fly to northern Queensland to do a five-day hike.

I am so heavy with sadness that I cry when I'm packing my bag, I cry on the plane, I cry as I strap on the pack before we get on a small boat to take us to the remote island where we are hiking.

I feel like I haven't stopped moving in months. Mystics and saints walked to find serenity. It is a sort of moving meditation, where stillness and nature combine. The hike will not be another gruelling task to complete, but rather a contemplative walk. I'm in a bad way – I'd never worked so hard, on something so incredibly unusual, difficult and high stakes, wanted something so fervently, and in the end failed in the endeavour.

I need the reality of the executions to settle somewhere, somehow, even though some part of me will never accept what has happened. I have to come down to some quiet place, where I can walk and not talk and let beautiful, wild nature start to work its healing magic.

Before I start the hike along the Thorsborne Trail on Hinchinbrook Island, I fit in a couple of small practice walks while the Mercy Campaign is in full swing. I trudge with a small pack and new boots on the stretch of car-heavy road that takes me from my home in Bellevue Hill to my office in Surry Hills. I carry a few heavy novels in my daypack.

As I will find out, this practice is woefully inadequate.

There are around ten of us doing the hike, travel journalists from around the world, many of whom have trekked some of the greatest and most difficult trails in the world. We walk along the beach on a bright, 30-degree autumn day, sand firm beneath our feet. Day one's walk is only 6.5 kilometres – nothing, right? I can do that in an hour or two, just like walking along the cliffs from Bondi to Bronte and back, or from La Trobe Street to the MCG.

My pack feels weird, though – a lot heavier than the practice pack I took along Oxford Street. In this pack I carry a tent, a sleeping bag, a mat, enough food for five days, clothes (including really bulky socks), toilet paper, two torches, a phone, a couple of chargers (including a battery one), lollies, snacks and three litres of water that comes from a weird bladder/hose thing that I keep in the top of my backpack to suck while walking. With its tube and bag, it looks alarmingly like something you'd wake up attached to after major surgery.

The other thing about my pack is that it is not actually my pack. It belongs to Patrick, who is taller than me, with broader shoulders. As we walk along that first sandy stretch it becomes apparent that, as well as being heavy, the pack is going to be a real irritant. The right shoulder strap keeps slipping off, unbalancing me, and the fidgeting and adjusting, the leaning forward and shifting of weight never really stops until I take the pack off – a pleasure so sublime that I actually moan with joy every time the load falls from my shoulders.

But before I can take the pack off, I have to walk. And after ten minutes of flat sand we get to the boulders – huge things that look like they've been hurled onto the beach by an angry god. Apart from swimming around them, the only way through is to climb over them, which doesn't seem right, as this is a hike, not a climb.

The others – those seasoned hiking journalists – leap from boulder to boulder before disappearing from sight. It's hours before I see them again.

I am slow. My legs aren't long enough and my arms aren't strong enough to negotiate the boulders with ease. To make matters worse, when I launch myself onto the next boulder and try to haul myself up it (grazing the insides of my arms), the weight of the pack and the loose straps pull me backwards, leading to the sensation that I am about to lose my grip, fall back and dash my head on the rocks below. When I am not trying to drag myself up the rocks, I am frozen in fear.

A couple of times I manage to take my pack off and hurl it up the rocks, so I don't tip backwards. Seeing I am struggling, the rangers we are travelling with position themselves above and below me. The one below grasps the back of my pack and shoves it forward, giving me upwards momentum. The other ranger, on the boulder above, grabs my hand and pulls me up.

This continues for another half-a-dozen boulders, until we get to an area that doesn't involve climbing; instead it involves walking across rocks of different sizes, surface areas and degrees of slipperiness.

Before the hike, I'd been warned by many that it wasn't the snakes or the crocodiles I needed to worry about, it was the small things – the twisted ankle, for example, caused by slipping in between the rocks. There is a lot on my mind during this hike but, walking over those rocks, everything becomes narrowed to a laser point. I am too focused on looking down to see the scenery, too focused on each step to think about anything else. It is like the purest form of meditation – but horrible.

On the boat on the way over, our skipper spoke about a woman who'd managed to call the mainland to be rescued because she'd had a sore foot during this hike. We on the boat hooted with derision, then wondered – isn't it a criminal offence to get rescued for a minor ailment?

On the first day, I am preoccupied with the heaviness of my pack. I'm huffing and puffing as I walk, and have a fear for most of the day that I will have a heart attack. The ranger behind me, Evan, tells me, 'It's going to be a struggle but we'll get there in the end.'

At the rest stop, the others take off up a hill where there is meant to be incredible views of the coastline. I rest, hurling the pack off in disgust. 'Fuck this shit,' I say. Bright blue and black butterflies circle us, round and round and round they go. They are preferable to the sandflies that bothered me as I walked along the beach.

Evan tells me that some people do the walk in a day. But 'three nights and four days is the most comfortable time'. He sits beside me and we eat some muesli bars and nuts. We've only been walking for an hour but I'm starving. The island has no shops so we had to bring in our food – bags of dehydrated, powdery stuff that is too bizarre to contemplate closely: lamb and red wine risotto, beef rendang, satay chicken, apple pie, yoghurt and muesli, all of it looking the same. Stopping at a clearing for lunch or dinner, we boil up water on stoves we brought in (no fires allowed), then put a bag in water for ten minutes. To open the package and look at the food while it is still in utero is to confront an existential horror – the lamb growing and expanding inside the bag, the colour and texture of cement, the risotto bloating but somehow not softening, and tasting of soil.

My fellow hikers compete with each other about whose meal is the most disgusting. Chicken tikka masala, roast beef and the cooked breakfast are frontrunners. The worst, though, is not finishing the meal and having to carry it, half-eaten, around in your pack due to the absence of bins on the island. I'll never forget the sensation of sticking my hand into my backpack in the middle of the night, reaching for toilet paper but instead groping the remnants of sausage and mash.

Somehow I manage to get through day one without dying, doing my ankle or collapsing from exhaustion. Stopping is the best bit. We camp at Little Ramsay Bay, on the beach. It is lovely, just like I imagined an island paradise to be. I even enjoy a furtive swim, despite the warnings that there are crocodiles in the region. Sitting on the beach as the sun goes down, we pass around a bag of goon, and stir our dinners in their little bags. I fall in a creek while filling my three-litre drink bottle with stagnant water that has algae floating in it. One of the other hikers has to put up my tent for me, as I'm too feeble and weak to stake the poles. I am asleep by 7pm but at around 3.45am I wake from a nightmare about jail cells and the jungle and midnight executions.

Day two is 10 kilometres, and the 'more difficult day', Evan says. And so it comes to pass. My pack is adjusted and I am strapped into it like an astronaut about to be launched into space. But the take-off, such as it is, is wobbly. As I set off, something is happening to my legs. They are like jelly. I quickly drop behind the group.

The two rangers stay with me, one closely behind me, one closely in front. There are many boulders to clamber over and the only way I can get through it is for someone behind me to boost, or sort of throw my pack forward, propelling me onto the next rock, while the ranger in front grabs my arm and hauls me up.

What is the point of this? I wonder, finding it impossible to take in the beauty of the island under such stressful circumstances. I am not anywhere near achieving my goal of serenity. There are scheduled stops at waterfalls and swimming holes. There are trees to sit under while drinking ginger wine and gazing up at butterflies. There are powdered beef satays to eat. But by mid-morning I have fallen well behind the other hikers, and don't even have time to stop for breaks. The rangers – who are walking slowly with me – become worried that we will be stuck out here at night. They've had slow walkers before – a group of elderly Indigenous women who were the area's native-title holders. They plodded along but eventually they made it to camp before dark. That is the crucial thing – to get to a safe place before dark.

The ground underneath us in the lower, more tropical parts of the island has a curious stench, one I have never smelt before. 'Excrement from carpet snakes,' a ranger explains.

On we walk until it becomes more like a march. The rangers fashion me a stick, which I use to heave myself up goat tracks and slow my progress as we go down the other side. When the path pitches steeply it sometimes feels safer to slide down the track on my backside. I am wearing my favourite orange yoga pants. The material ladders as I slide down rocks.

The creek crossings are the worst. I fall in maybe six creeks, sometimes multiple falls each creek – to the front, to the side, on my back, getting wet, cut and bruised, my lower lip trembling as I almost but don't quite cry. Walking through the jungle I can feel my chest tightening and my breath becoming shallow. Is this it? Heart attack time? My friend Erik walked the Kokoda Track and two men in his group died of heart failure while hiking. My chest tightens even more, the prospect of a heart attack creating further anxiety.

Maybe it's simple biomechanics and my straps are too tight. But if I loosen my pack it pulls me backwards, and that could result in me falling and hitting my head and dying. The rangers would have to stay with my body until daybreak, then climb a peak and signal a passing ship ...

The rangers – tough Queenslanders who know and love this island – walk ahead, cutting through the thicker areas with machetes. The conversation keeps my mind off the inevitable heart attack: we talk about the cultural relativism of female genital mutilation and witch burning in Papua New Guinea, whether people in cities are unfriendly compared with country people, what happens to the people who wander off-track and get lost. I like them a lot and can't help but feel guilty about what a drain I am on their resources. They are now hobbling a little as well, after being forced to walk so slowly (it's apparently harder on the body to walk slowly than it is to walk fast).

Finally we arrive at a beach. Surely this is the end? Dark is falling. I am bent over my stick, like I am a crippled ninety-year-old.

My socks and pants are soaked from falling in the creek. My back hurts. Everything hurts.

The other hikers, who have had a lovely break for a few hours at a waterfall, put up my tent. I collapse inside without any supper. Day three is meant to be harder still. The rangers are worried. Can I complete day three? The various falls into different creeks have had a cumulative effect.

A ranger comes into my tent at 3am. Due to the weather and the currents, there is only a small window of time to contact Search and Rescue. Can I keep hiking? Can I make it across the boulders and down the creeks that await tomorrow? Can I get up from where I have sort of collapsed in fetal position, too tired to even remove my muddy hiking clothes? If not, I will need to be rescued.

Around 4am a distress call is placed to the sea rescue crew on the mainland. The forecast is for rough seas, and there are only a few hours around dawn when it will be safe enough for a vessel to rescue me.

I pack all my things back in the enormous, hated backpack. I smash and mash up the tent in the bag. It doesn't matter now – I won't be using it again. I don't know where the rescuers will take me or what will happen when I get there. I have no money or ID or wallet. They are locked in the ranger's car in the town of Cardwell.

I walk down to the beach in the weak pre-dawn light. Everything looks watery and unreal, like an impressionist painting seen from a dirty window. I wait to hear the motor of the boat chopping through the water. I am sore and ashamed, like maybe I only deserve to be rescued if something massive, bloody and bad happened to me – a leg bitten off by a crocodile, for instance, or an actual heart attack, rather than some falls and an anxiety attack.

I sit on a big rock facing the heaving sea and watch the sun come up. It is the first time I have stopped and looked up. This corner of the world really is beautiful.

**

Hiking is enjoying something of a moment. It's not simply exercise, but also a tonic for your soul. Just look at Cheryl Strayed's bestselling hiking memoir, *Wild* (and the Reese Witherspoon film that followed). She shot heroin the night before she started hiking, and in the hard graft of the walk, she worked her life out.

The narrative creeping into hiking is something different from the daggy bushwalking tropes from the '70s and '80s, something our fathers and mothers with their long socks and tins of insect repellent and non-hiking boots (indeed their lack of any expensive kit) wouldn't necessarily recognise. It's not just the hero's journey – human versus the elements. It's the metaphysical aspect of hiking, the fact that when you walk, you work things out, that things become unknotted. The longer and harder the track, the more your physical labours will start healing the wounds that might lie in your soul. To stay at home, watch television or sleep is to fester or remain inert. To walk, particularly to walk hard somewhere isolated, is to take action, to somehow beat the thing inside you.

What does it mean, then, to be beaten by a hike? (Or rather to be beaten by yourself, unprepared for the hike.) People who go on these things are meant to return triumphant – sore but elated by a sense of accomplishment. I return feeling embarrassment and shame.

I'm discharged from the hospital without any money or ID. After a few phone calls some very kind people at a motel in Lucinda agree to take me in until the group returns. I stay in my room during the day and read, scratching my sandfly bites, and drink wine with the motel owners at night. They've had interesting lives: a rancher in Texas, a cardiac nurse in Brisbane. They try to make me feel better by saying, 'Well, I couldn't do that walk.'

Two days later the group returns after completing the hike and they tell me that day three wasn't too hard and day four was a short dawdle down the beach. 'You could have made it,' they say.

I return to Sydney to a massive ambulance bill and regular physiotherapy sessions, and the sense that serenity doesn't always appear after a struggle. And you can't always work things out by walking.

*

The years dissolve as quickly as sugar in hot tea, and by 2016 I am still searching for serenity. But after the terrible hike, it has become a more gentle search – enjoyable even. There is no rush, I think in my more Zen moments, it will unfurl and unfold for me in exactly the way it is meant to. I'm doing Vedic meditation most days, which helps. When I get into a routine with it, I feel like it is giving me that *peace the world cannot provide*. But I'm curious to see what else is out there.

I keep coming across the writing and the teaching of the same cadre of spiritual writers. But none seem as prolific as Deepak Chopra – an author, public speaker and all-round New Age modern guru who's been around *forever*. He's written more than eighty books and is frequently on television. His appearances on *Oprah* made him a household name. At almost seventy he is one of the wealthiest and most successful figures in the alternative medicine scene. He is wellness personified. So when I hear he's coming to Melbourne to give a weekend seminar, I'm curious.

I want to unpack Deepak, so to speak.

I don't know what to expect at the live event, but I'm surprised that it's this low-key. The crowd is in the hundreds, not the thousands, and they are subdued and focused. Chopra himself is understated, the cadence, volume and pace of his voice unchanging – soporific, even.

At the more tent revival–style events, the perfect pause, the dramatic emphasis, is everything. It whips up the crowd and lets them know that if they send POSITIVE AFFIRMATIONS – YES! AFFIRMATIONS! – TO THEIR CELLS, THEY. WILL. LIVE ... FOREVER! (And the crowd goes wild.)

But Deepak Chopra, veteran of thousands of public appearances, is not a pulse-raiser. For the whole two days it's just him on a bare stage with a screen at the Melbourne Convention Centre, talking in a monotone, covering a vast amount of ground, from how to slow the ageing process to how to have more interesting dreams.

This is New Age lite, suburban spirituality – the pack of angel cards on the mantelpiece next to the Pixie portraits of the grandkids, the consulting of newspaper horoscopes. And this being Melbourne, and winter, most people are dressed in black puffer jackets and big scarves – a group that could have been scooped up at random from Chadstone Shopping Centre.

I'm here with two friends, all of us Chopra first-timers. They went to the Melbourne Convention Centre last year to hear the Dalai Lama speak and the vibe was 'very different', my friend Sophie says.

'Lots of Tibetan prayer flags, and all these colours ...', says her sister.

'People wearing hemp.'

'Monks.'

'Dreadlocks.'

'People looked like they were really living it.'

No one here looks like they are living it – this is spirituality sotto voce.

'I'm going to be talking about almost every aspect of healing,' Chopra tells us from the unadorned stage. He's wearing black pants and a sleeveless jacket, with bright-red sneakers. His glasses have diamonds embedded in the arms. Chopra is in Australia to promote his 'six pillars of wellbeing': sleep; meditation and stress management; exercise; healthy emotions like love, compassion and joy; peace of mind; and good nutrition and hydration. All sensible stuff.

He starts off talking about the healing power of sleep, 'a fundamental pillar of wellbeing'. It's hard to argue with this. I've had particular trouble sleeping and am now getting ill. I sit down the back of the auditorium, my body racked with coughs, my 'area' a mess of tissues and water bottles.

Sleeping is the most efficient way to improve health, he says. It will 'aid in the elimination of toxins, provide order from chaos, encourage renewal and repair, increase immunity, memory, unconscious processing and creativity' – among other things. 'Ask yourself any question before you sleep and it will be processed in sleep and you will get the answer in the morning.'

So far, so good. But then Chopra goes off-piste, and all 'science-y', talking about his new book, *Super Genes*. Chopra reckons 95 per cent of disease-related gene mutations are influenced by how we think, how we feel, and our relationships. In other words – we make ourselves sick. And not just sick – but terminally ill.

A few years earlier, at a meditation centre in Ubud (just before my disastrous 'healing' session with Riki), I met a group of women who were all on the alternative healing circuit. My curiosity was piqued – they looked less *Eat, Pray, Love*, than suburban mums who had got on the wrong plane and ended up on the wrong holiday.

Over dinner, I discovered that three of them had cancer and one had Parkinson's. They were sick, but well enough to travel. They had a window of time, a grace period, and they were spending it in Bali.

They had read Deepak Chopra and motivational author Louise Hay, and over dinner they told me how they had caused their own illnesses. This was not through lifestyle choices that we associate with cancer – they were not smokers, and were only occasional drinkers – instead it was their emotions that had caused their cancer. Their anger. Their repressed sexual drives. Their unexplored trauma, going back to when they were girls. All the things they could have been but weren't. All the things they could have said but didn't. These things caused their cancer, *were* their cancer.

Pad Thai and pots of ginger tea. The heat and wetness of the night and the beads of sweat on the bottles of mineral water and the driver booked the next day to take them to the place in the countryside where someone they called a healer would, manually and in a machine, shake the cancer out of them in eight-hour stretches. I argued with them, like Robin Williams does with Matt Damon in *Good Will Hunting*: 'It's not your fault, it's not your fault, it's not your fault.' The bill came, my case doomed – they weren't even listening. They had read the books and listened to the tapes and this was their firm belief. But to me it seemed like just another way of being a woman, another way of blaming and hating yourself, of giving yourself the smallest lamb chop, of not making a fuss, of the quiet voice saying again, as it's always said, 'Sorry, it's my fault.' Or maybe it's just that we need to tell ourselves a story. A rogue cell dividing and dividing and dividing and dividing and dividing does not in itself a good story make.

Chopra does not move explicitly into this dark territory over the weekend but it's a philosophy coded into much of his materials. Pacing the stage, he tells us, '95 per cent of your genes can be influenced by you – your consciousness, your being, your soul. By changing the activity, you can change your body – and this is related to how we age and how we get sick.'

'Awareness is the key to transformation and reinventing the body,' he says. And the key to this key is affirmations, which involve repeating a positive mantra or expression until it sort of 'seeps' into your body. The affirmation that Chopra recommends is: 'Every day in every way I am increasing my physical and mental capacity. My biological set point is …' and at this point he tells us to pick a number. 'If you are sixty, make it forty; if you are forty, make it twenty. Go back fifteen or twenty years. Don't make it zero – you'll disappear into an orgasm.'

Everyone laughs, a little grossed out. But I am confused, as if I've walked in on a physics lecture when I am meant to be in a politics class. It doesn't make sense. Do our bodies really behave this way? Can we really influence the behaviour of our genes? Affirmations don't sound like they'd really cut the mustard. Aren't they just words said to ourselves in a mirror? Prayers to a nameless god about how we wish things could be?

The next question is from a woman who stands up and asks, 'I arrived from Singapore last night and I couldn't sleep, even though I was very tired. Why is that?'

'Your mind was too busy – you were anticipating this. We'll get to sleep later,' says Chopra, referring to the subject matter of sleep, not saying that the woman would literally 'get to sleep later'.

The next question is 'Can your brain heal lesions?'

'Yes, you can regulate the body and brain – we'll get to that later.'

Later in the day, a neurologist who also teaches yoga asks Chopra a question. I am intrigued that a member of the medical community is engaging with the New Age. Via another audience member, I pass a note to the neurologist after the tea break. *You're really interesting*, I write. *I like your question. Let's talk.*

He rings me at the end of day one. 'What did you think of today?' I ask him.

'It was good,' he says. 'What Chopra has done is distil a lot of the knowledge from the Veda [a large body of texts originating in India and mostly published in Sanskrit]. He's distilled the lessons from the top hundred or so texts and presents them in his own way to a Western audience.'

So this is nothing new.

In the lunch break the following day people start queuing up to have their book signed by Chopra. I ask one woman, Sharon, why she is here. 'My mum had one of his books. I read it and it opened my eyes to the idea that this' – she gestures to the half-empty lobby of the convention centre – 'is not all there is to the world. There's something else.'

Chopra himself says, 'Most people are not alive – they are walking around in sleep, like in a computer program. We need to wake up to the fact that we are living consciousness that is destined to have an infinity of experience.'

I leave Chopra's event early, very much feeling like I am walking around in sleep. I check in to my hotel in Fitzroy, turn on the bar heater and by 6pm I am in bed. I lie there feeling mortal, helpless and ill, and try to remember the mantra Chopra taught us to stop the ageing process.

It's a nice fairytale before I go to sleep.

The year I see Deepak, 2016, I step up my search for serenity – in part because I am researching this book, but also because I still haven't quite got there. I'm after a way to balance the hedonism that I love and the serenity that I crave. Is there a way to make them co-exist? For so many people it's an all-or-nothing thing. They shun all partying as a gateway for toxins and the road away from wellness that leads to ruin. In this world, hedonism is seen in moral terms – it is bad, and to succumb to life's base pleasures is to show a moral weakness. But I am looking for a way to integrate (that word again) the two – to party and celebrate when the mood takes me, and also be serene and able to go inwards. Do they have to be mutually exclusive?

Apparently not, as I'd find out in Thailand.

Via word of mouth I book into a rustic utopia that takes more than a day to get to. You can fast while you're there, or take any number of alternative healing workshops. Or you can just sit in the bar all day and drink Bintang, then head to the beach at night for parties that go until dawn.

It's a ridiculous and wonderful place all at the same time. In the cafe on the first day, while drinking a thick vegetable juice and sweating profusely, I eavesdrop on two men, one Australian and the other English, both in their thirties.

'I had Shiva come and speak to me for six hours and guide my meditation – and Shiva would just be saying, "Love your body,"' says the English guy in the sort of faded voice you get when you've been fasting and feel really weak. He has a shaved head and small John Lennon glasses, with beads looped around his neck.

The humidity is high, the sea is flat and there is no breeze. A ceiling fan chops at the thick air with little effect.

The Australian guy sitting across from him is shirtless, with a thin, toned body, high hair and red string wristbands. He's sipping a carrot juice and making 'yeah, uh-huh' noises.

'And then I would be in thoughts and memories and Shiva would say again, "Love your body." Six hours and I connected with the masculine archetype and now with the masculine/feminine thing as well and I feel safe with it, and it takes me to the place I need to go.'

'Yeah, uh-huh.'

'One time he took me to the lower chakras and that's where hell is. He said, "I can take you there," and I was just being lazy and unfocused, and I was like, "No, Shiva, I don't have to go there."'

'Yeah, uh-huh.'

Since the 1990s this place has evolved from a backpacker's hot tip to a place where hedge-fund dudes, Silicon Valley types and Bondi trustafarians drop in for weeks and months to live the good life. The good life is a beguiling mix and muddle of wellness and hedonism that somehow holds the contradiction in place without missing a step. Here you can party all night in the jungle, drink delicious cocktails, eat cake and then switch into detox mode with healthy juices, massage, yoga classes and fasting.

'You go and just connect,' the general manager tells me when I pull up on the sand with a suitcase and order a beer. We are sitting at a table facing the darkening sea. He takes his two peace fingers and points them at me. 'Connect.'

'On drugs?'

'No, there's no drugs here. Through the eyes, you have a connection with people.'

I sign up for ecstatic dance, thinking of Gloria's Sufi dancing in Bali, and how some cultures believe that serenity comes not through stillness but through movement. At dusk I make my way along the trail. Backing onto the jungle, the hall is all lit up with fairy lights. There are around eight of us and we all sit in a circle, with Darren as our guide. He is Australian, from a small town outside Sydney, and has hair so blond it's almost white. He wears those Thai fisherman's pants with the complicated knotting at the front and more billows than a bagpipe – yet he carries it off. He has a sort of regal bearing.

'I take people into the jungle and we do ancestral movement and games,' he explains. 'Everything in the jungle speaks to us. I'm interested in rewilding the human being.'

Darren has gone into the jungle earlier in the day and picked mushrooms. They are mixed up in a murky brown drink in the middle of the circle. I am not sure if the mushrooms are hallucinogenic or if they are just *mushroom* mushrooms. Music is playing. It sounds vaguely tribal. Darren passes around the drink and asks us to say what we are grateful for. There are several fasters in the group whose gratitude seems deeper and more profound than the gratitude of the other people (the eaters), who stick with banal statements such as 'I am grateful to be here'. The fasters are grateful not just for being here, but also for being. In the darkened room, the whites of their eyes are illuminated like they're wearing novelty contact lenses. Their number includes a hypnotist, a lawyer and a traveller who had previously worked in the arts and culture sector in Darwin.

Over the next ninety minutes we lose ourselves in an ecstatic dance, starting with all these Polynesian-style movements and clapping, then call and response, and then, after an hour, once I drop into it, I am dancing in my sweat-soaked, now yellowing white linen shirt. Massive Attack is playing and then Kanye, and Darren plays African drums and guitar and then a flute and we all lie on yoga mats and the candles around the room burn and sharp yelps come from the jungle, and the mushroom drink, if it has any effect, is to make everything smooth and even and lush and just-right – serene, even. This feeling lasts for a while after the music stops, then there's a spoken word bit; this guy comes on, speaking in an Indian accent and sounding very far away and mellow, saying, 'Be grateful for everything. Be grateful for everything.'

I think of all the varied, gorgeous surfaces on the Earth I have walked in the search for serenity and I murmur, 'I am, dude, I am.'

Then one day, I get a call. It's a fellow journalist. He has a challenge for me. Would I sign up to an intensive, week-long group psychotherapy retreat in the bush?

'You've done a lot of travel journalism,' he says. 'Think of it as an incredible, wild, sometimes scary but hugely rewarding journey, but the journey is not to another country, it's into yourself.'

'Wot?' I say. 'That sounds kind of awful.'

My passport is full of stamps. I am constantly leaving and arriving. The departure board at the airport flickers and updates and flickers and changes, even in my dreams. I'm greedy to see it all. Yet a journey of the internal kind? It scares me. This promises to be different from the other retreats I've done. It promises to be more intense and to go deeper. It seems an edgier, more dangerous road. There is to be no yoga, no oms or incense – instead we will be working with our own dark material. It's called Path of Love.

Do I want to go there? Not really. But … maybe it is time. I am curious about what I might find. Maybe serenity, finally?

So after thinking about it for, like, ten minutes, I sign up.

Almost everyone I know is against me going on this retreat. It freaks people out more than when I went on the multi-day hike while emotionally fragile and physically unprepared. Friends pensively riff on the theme of 'don't change' or 'don't let them change you'. I meet my boss Emily from the *Guardian* for a drink at Circular Quay the day before I go 'in'.

'You know you don't have to do it if you don't want to,' she says. We are drinking good sparkling wine and the good harbour is sparkling before us. Why disturb the universe when it's all humming along nicely? 'Make sure they don't take your phone, in case it's dreadful and you need to ring and get someone to pick you up.' She's had to rescue me from stories before. She's called me back from swimming in shark-infested waters, from hospital beds in Far North Queensland and all manner of strife closer to home.

Apart from one couple who did a workshop called the Hoffman Process, none of my friends have done any self-development courses. It's uncharted territory. And if they have done it, they've kept quiet about it. There is scepticism – and a degree of disapproval.

'I won't change,' I promise people before I go in. Yet I get the sense that whatever happens in there, I won't stay the same.

I am met at a lonely country station by a Path of Love volunteer, who drives me and three other participants to the retreat centre in the Hunter Valley. One participant, a woman in her sixties, is particularly garrulous, talking at speed about the treatment of refugees on Manus Island and Nauru, and then some dude or thing called Osho. What is Osho? It sounds like a clothing label. The rest of us are mostly silent – jaws set at a certain point of tension, eyes out the window as the landscape rushes past: scraggly ghost gums, the shapes of kangaroos in the mid-distance, the sky a crinkly blue, a thicket of trees whose highest points bend into each other like a bush cathedral.

So what is the Path of Love? It's a global phenomenon, with retreats in North and South America, Europe, the Middle East and Australia. The vibe is a mix of Eastern spirituality and Western psychotherapy, drawing on the works of Sufi mystics, Jung, the teachings of Buddha and Jesus, the cartoons of Michael Leunig and the writings of Irish poet and philosopher John O'Donohue. And Osho.

I later find out that Osho is not a clothing label (although you can get Osho T-shirts and other branded products). He is a big deal, a crazy controversial spiritual guru formerly known as the Bhagwan Shree Rajneesh. He was an Indian spiritual teacher in the 1960s and '70s, and later in the US, where his teachings commanded huge – rapt – audiences. He had the largest collection of Rolls Royces in the world, and preached sexual liberation and materialism. But he also believed that every human was his or her own god, and had within them the divine. Science and spirituality should both be embraced; they were not exclusive. And also this – life should be fun. There is no god other than life itself.

Osho died aged fifty-eight in 1990. Some of his teachings are carried on today, at a centre in Pune, and with strains of his work running through the Path of Love workshops.

Established in 1996 and running in Australia for twenty years, the Path of Love can loosely be described as a self-development course. In Australia, it's run by Alima Cameron and Samved Dass, who have worked in counselling and psychotherapy for more than thirty years. They spent time around Osho in the early wild days.

People come to it by word of mouth, often when facing a cri-sis – stress, a bereavement, unhappiness or anxiety. But some come just out of curiosity or a desire to explore aspects of themselves that have been cut off or repressed over time. 'They are seeking a wider view on what life is,' says Samved.

Participants are screened via an interview and a fairly exhaus-tive and probing questionnaire. 'People need to have a certain ability to move and need to be psychologically stable enough to do the work,' says Samved. 'People need to have a degree of functionality.' The work we will be doing is emotionally dif-ficult – and physical. You need to be strong to get through it, although there is a lot of support. It's very well run and organ-ised and there is a large staff – a ratio of almost one to one during much of the week.

There are around thirty participants who will be doing the week-long course with me. They are mostly Australian but some have come from other parts of the world especially for this course, which is run here twice a year. Our ages range from thirties to six-ties, although Samved tells me that people in their twenties right through to their eighties have completed the Path of Love.

At the start of the week, we are encouraged to leave our outside life at the door. Phones and iPads are collected with the promise that they'll be returned to us at the end of the week (I don't hand mine in – but I cannot get signal out here). We then sit in a small-ish seminar room and wait for our facilitators. There is a palpable air of fear. Some people are sort of sniffling or quietly crying and I'm immediately freaked out. *Why are they crying?* It hasn't even started yet. There are boxes of tissues at various intervals around the room. It's human nature to turn your attention to people who are crying, and I try to look around discreetly. I'm scared. Maybe I should leave now, before it's too late.

Then it's too late.

Samved and Alima come in and congratulate us on the brave decision to do the program (there is nervous laughter at this) and then take us through some of the central tenets that we are to keep returning to over the course of the week. These are things such as 'I am willing to face where I am afraid' and 'I am willing to really look at what is missing in my life'. There are rules. We will be on time for all sessions. We will not use stimulants. We will not be violent to ourselves or each other. We will not have sex with anyone while we are here (or any participants or helpers for three months after we leave).

While I'm here to write a story, I also think it will be a good opportunity to turn over a few things in my life and look at them from different angles. There are some 'areas' where I need to clean up my act. There are patterns and habits and beliefs that I hold that no longer serve me. I try not to feel too scared about how exposed I will feel, picking up these rocks of mine and watching spiders crawl out. Or how defensive I'll feel when others pick up those rocks, or how vulnerable I'll feel with others watching all my spiders scuttle out. I tell myself I'm lucky to have this opportunity to take a week to look deeply and fully at my life and pull it apart. *This won't hurt a bit*, I think, knowing that it's not true.

It's getting dark now and a north wind is blowing. We are led into a hall and divided into three groups of around ten people each. I take them all in quickly – their faces are blank, some smile (but they are nervous so it looks like rictus), others keep their eyes to the ground. Everyone in my group seems to be in their thirties and forties. There's a mix of men and women. Some wear wedding bands. Some look exhausted. No one appears to be what you would call 'relaxed'. Everyone is wearing the clothes we were asked to wear: comfortable, loose, exercise-y gear that can withstand a lot of movement.

First we must each stand up and tell the group why we are here (a story about what's going on, what's gone wrong) and that we are committed to change. Others in the group are meant to stand up in support when they get a sense of the person's commitment and authenticity. I don't really want to expose myself to a bunch of strangers. There are dissatisfactions and disappointments in my life that I can barely admit to myself, let alone to people I have just met. And this commitment to change . . . that sounds kind of hard.

When it's my turn, I stand up and babble a bit about why I am committed to the process that we are about to undertake. When others have stood up to speak through their tears, snot and terror, it's only been a few minutes before we have all been standing in solidarity. But I've been talking for ten minutes or more and no one is standing up. I'm getting desperate. I've run out of things to share. *Stand up, you fuckers*, I think, and possibly say. *Stand up.* I have nothing left to say, so I just stand there in front of the group and shrug. I couldn't feel more exposed if I had completely stripped off my clothes. *Stand up, you fuckers.*

Usually I love speaking in front of groups of people I don't know. My ideal audience is five or six. I'm good with glib jokes and anecdotes. But none of it works here. The members of the group are stony faced.

I take another breath and dig deep and say the first thing that comes to my head. It probably emerges confused and garbled, but I'm so obviously uncomfortable that it transmits as authentic. One by one the group stand up, and, traumatised, I'm released from the stage. I feel like sobbing from relief.

We are then told to get close to each other and gravitate towards someone we feel a connection with. They are to be our 'buddy' for the week. I gravitate towards a younger, good-looking guy with puppy-dog eyes. Familiar terrain. I can't help myself – even here.

In the next round of 'sharing' we have to stand up and people in the group say what they think of you. 'We all have our conditioned personality, which is set up by all the pain from our childhood,' says Samved. 'We put on our personality mask and that is obscuring our ability to be natural and relaxed.'

To be relaxed is the optimum state, I will find. Not happy, not joyful, not bouncing off the walls – what we are really aiming for is to be *relaxed*. But to get to relaxed is not relaxing. In order to remove our masks, first the mask has to be identified. Man, this is the *worst*. Members of the group stand up in front of us and we have to say what we think of them. I only have first impressions of these people, in an artificially intense, intimate and stressful space. So one by one the strangers around me stand up, nervous and afraid, and I and the others volunteer assessments such as 'you have sad eyes' or 'you have low self-esteem' or some other statement informed by the thinnest of thin slicing. Really, what do I know of these people – or anyone? And what do they know of me?

I wait almost until the end. Then it is my turn to stand up.

My level of discomfort during this exercise is so deep, I can barely take in what people are saying. One guy tells me I have trouble making eye contact. I immediately get self-conscious and self-correct by staring at him, before getting uncomfortable and looking away. Why have I not been told this before? Does that mean I've been going around *all my life* not looking at people in the eye?

One woman says I have a problem 'committing to commitment'. Yeah, that's probably true. I always like to keep my options open. Another says, 'You're afraid to spend time with yourself.' I nod, while thinking, *That's not true – I'm a writer, I spend huge slabs of time alone. Right? Right?* Some of the 'feedback' is old news. Yes, I live life with my head, not my heart. And, yes, I am my own worst critic. But the mask I'm wearing is slipping down.

It's only day one and already I'm feeling big emotions – mostly fear and vulnerability. But that is what the process promised: they would take us down from our heads to our hearts, and the best way of doing this is to think less and feel more.

It's late now, and I feel drained. Alima asks us to close our eyes. *Oh, what now?* But her words are reassuring, almost like a mother's to a frightened child: 'You are meant to be here and there is no other place you need to be right now. You've paid your money, got on a plane, got here. And now you are here. Let it all unfold as it will.'

It's the verbal equivalent of having your forehead stroked.

As we leave the hall with our buddies (mine loops his arm through mine, like we are schoolchildren), I notice many people walking back to their cabins in tears.

In trying to dodge unpleasant feeling we often numb ourselves or distract ourselves. We don't even know we are doing it. There's no social media or smart phones or booze around this week. Without distractions, the feelings will have their week in the sun.

During the week I get a lot of insights around this. Unconsciously I blunt my feelings through drinking, distractions such as the internet or television or social media. I dull them through prescription drugs that promise to take away sadness and anxiety. We don't even realise it, but so much of the time we walk around numb. It's just as Deepak and others have said.

Our minds work hard to label our experiences and feelings as good, bad, fun, boring, etc. – so a lot of what we experience is filtered through a judgemental lens. What I have been taught from Matt and Aruna, and now here, is to let the feelings run through me without putting a name on them, without labelling them as good or bad or whatever. The feelings will eventually run their course and be replaced by other feelings. There's no point getting too attached to them. The trick is just to loosen the reins a bit and, as the Tame Impala song goes, just let it happen.

To move into a state where feelings have primacy over thinking, the Path of Love has a number of elements that are quite physical – sensual even (not to be confused with sexual). Touch plays a big part, as distinct from most traditional therapy set-ups, which are very much hands off.

On the first day I wake early (my bed is very soft, maybe too soft), even before someone walks around outside playing chimes from 5.30am. We're to start the day with an hour-long meditation called Dynamic. My roommate and I are not meant to talk outside the sessions but in the drowsy pre-dawn we compare notes. She is cool – a doctor and mother of five who has been here before.

'What is Dynamic?' I ask. We have not been told what is going to happen. (Samved later tells me why people aren't told what happens before they go in – they are liable to get scared and not do the program in the first place.)

She shudders. 'Dynamic is awful.'

We walk down to the hall and I stand at the back while the drum and bass music gets progressively louder. Someone speaks into a microphone like a DJ at a rave.

Because I'm not properly prepared for it, when people start doing primal screaming, I freak the fuck out. I'm not used to people making loud sounds. Screaming is something I've reserved for when someone is actually *murdering* me. No wonder this retreat is miles from anywhere.

There are people doing 'grrrrrr' sounds (popular with men), or shrieking like they have lost a child (women), or moaning like they have been kicked in the balls or womb. It is too loud and too intense and I don't like it. For a while I curl up in a ball and put my hands over my ears and wait for it to pass. I try to join in but all I can muster is a couple of low-level moans, like I am suffering bad period pain. Nothing is coming to the surface. I look around and notice a couple of other women curled up and holding their ears. My roommate looks as if she has gone 'vacant': there in body but sort of mentally checked out. I vow to find the scream-resisters later and talk about how we could get out of Dynamic. The next bit of this Sufi-style meditation involves jumping up and down for fifteen minutes. It's meant to awaken the sex drive. Jumping like this hurts my boobs, though. I also feel self-conscious even though no one is looking at me. I should have packed a sports bra.

When I ask one of the facilitators later why we start the day with such vigorous – and unusual – physical activity, he tells me that it helps dislodge feelings that have been suppressed or buried in the body. Already, before breakfast, my Fitbit shows I've done more than 12,000 steps.

After an hour, when the meditation is over, the bush has that lovely early-morning glow, where even the harshest landscapes are bathed in a forgiving light. It has rained overnight. Dew sits heavy on the leaves, poised – ready to drop.

In the group sessions today I make a real effort to make eye contact with people. But it is a really sad and gruelling day. People stand up and talk about what is going on for them and it is wrenching. For the sake of their privacy I'll not say anything more about the others.

I stand up, clear my throat and talk about boys.

One of the facilitators, a big, masculine dude, stands up with a punching bag and kickboxing pads and tells me to hit him. As instructed, I run up to him in front of the group and give him a kick in the balls area, very hard, and scream, '*Fuck you!*' I do this several times and feel better but also physically exhausted.

In the afternoon we dance for hours. It's like a rave but without drugs or alcohol. We are encouraged to dance with our eyes closed. I keep opening mine and peering around at what everyone is doing until one of the helpers spots me and comes around with a blindfold. Then I'm dancing in the dark.

At certain points of the dance, people scream and cry and yell – just like they do in the morning, but it's less contained now. They are really letting it rip. My writer's mind is leaping out of my head; I'm imagining all the stories and things that happened to these people to make them howl with such pain and rage. The facilitator comes over to me with the punching bag again and tells me to 'let it out', which I do, and I begin to howl too. I would find the next day that I have actually screamed so hard, my voice is going.

On day three I sleep in and miss Dynamic – which, as you can imagine, is devastating. My 'buddy' is meant to report me missing, but thankfully he doesn't. I feel slow and drowsy. The process is taking it out of me. It's all that jumping and dancing and listening and emoting and processing. An article about the Path of Love in the UK *Sunday Times* talks about how much people eat – which I understand now. Meals – meant to be eaten in silence – are a process of refuelling. We're shovelling it down. The *Sunday Times* article also says a week at this retreat is the equivalent of going to therapy weekly for two years.

In the hall I hear the sound of screaming. My roommate joins me on the balcony in the morning sun. She snacks on some gluten-free crackers and tells me that the staff are doing their own process when we have our breaks.

The interesting principle at work is release and containment. You release whatever emotions need an outlet – old hurts, betrayals, ugly feelings – but you are doing it in a safe place, where you can spill out and rage and cry and there is no one judging you – in fact, they're encouraging you. I've never seen so many people in tears. Even when we are sitting quietly before sessions there is the sound of people sobbing around me. But I realise many participants feel relieved that they are in a place where they can just totally let go and let the tears flow. After all, if you walk down the street wailing and crying and screaming and beating things up with a rubber bat (we do that too), you would likely be committed.

Here, people come and hold you when you are crying. They stroke your feet and your hair. Sometimes you find yourself, when a slow song comes on, dancing in someone's arms. It is a helper. You are blindfolded and can't tell which one, and even if you could, it wouldn't really matter. Your head is on someone's chest and there is an eerie old Peter Gabriel song playing and the heart beating in their chest fills your eardrum, the temperature of your skin and their skin running hot.

By the end of the week, I get to recognise where people are in the room not by the sound of their voice, but by the sound of their weeping.

✳

Despite all the sound and fury, at this stage I still feel like I'm not going too deep. I'm yet to cry. Even though I shouldn't, I feel vaguely competitive with all the criers. They are really going for it, getting bang for their buck. And me? Is there nothing to feel sad about, or am I highly repressed? I begin to get stressed that my sorrow is so deep that it is at a place I can't access. Or that there is no sorrow, which means I am an unfeeling monster.

Through waking up the body, the process is supposed to quiet the mutinous mind. We are kept so busy with activities and sensations and stimuli that the mind has no chance to analyse anything we do. My mind, however, conducts its mutiny late at night. In the narrow single bed, with hot February winds blowing up the hill through the ghost gums and nothing but a noisy plastic fan for relief, my mind won't slow. It runs so fast, as if fast-forwarding through a tape, and plays a bizarre loop of Joe Hockey talking about the 2014 Federal Budget, over and over. Why? Who knows? But a surge of feelings, electrical in its currents and power, has short-circuited my thoughts, producing loops and jump cuts and nonsensical montages like a bad art installation, like a waking dream. It is only my exhausted and sore body that, night after night, manages to drag me to sleep.

**

After Dynamic on the third day Samved tells us it's Shame and Shadow Day, and my heart sinks. One of Carl Jung's major archetypes was the Shadow Self. There's the Persona, or mask, and alongside that is the Shadow, comprising repressed ideas, instincts, impulses, weaknesses, desires, perversions and embarrassing fears. The Shadow can be a source of creative energy, but it's mainly tied up with shame. The aim of today, Samved tells us, is not to purge the Shadow Self, but to bring it out into the light and somehow integrate it with the rest of our being. A sort of cold, whole-body shiver moves over me, like a sudden storm.

I'm not the only one who feels this way – the whole atmosphere in the room changes; atoms and air rearrange around this new charge.

This will be heavy. And so it proves to be.

When we file into the hall, Nirvana's 'Come as You Are' is blasting and I feel physically ill. I try to think what I can bring to the group that I've never told anyone, the thing I have gone to the greatest lengths to conceal. I have no shame.

Then I give it some thought. I have so much shame. The challenge will be picking what story of shame to share. So much, so much, so much, so much shame.

I try to imagine what shame others in the group will bring and brace myself. I also feel a pre-emptory compassion for my fellow group members and the things they're going to share today.

Shame and Shadow Day turns out to be very hard and cathartic, and once I get through it, I feel lighter and free – as if I've made some dangerous crossing (at night, headlamps bright then dim, carrying all my bags through a rising and dark river and the knotted and sharp foothills of a mountain – and on and on, walking carefully in the dark, looking at my feet, until it is safe and I can place the bags down. I have crossed, and I can continue my journey but it is lighter now, and I am unencumbered).

Later it is back to hitting the guy with the boxing pads. And then in the afternoon, in the special disco, I am hitting and hitting and hitting, long after everyone has stopped and is lying on their individual mattresses on the ground, heaving, sobbing, sighing and spent. My eye mask is slipping off and my dress is soaked with sweat. This is a workout for my inner life, and the energy I am producing has the force of a geyser. It is coming from a well somewhere within and the process has finally unleashed it – and it feels like it will never stop. I keep hitting and hitting and hitting.

On the evening of the third day there's a full moon and the bush is still and hot. It's meant to be a scorcher tomorrow, a total fire ban. The music – party music like Rihanna and Katy Perry – is blasting and we're all dancing together and swapping partners with a kind of abandon and swagger and swing. I'm dancing with men and women – people I've never met and people I know and people whose secrets I've heard (and they have heard mine). With these people, even though it's only been three days, I feel so warm and close, and kind too. I let them get into my space, all up close, our noses touching in a dance. It's joyous. I want to break eye contact at two seconds in but I try not to. Why is it so hard? It feels too intimate, like I am being too intrusive by staring. Breaking eye contact feels like giving the other person privacy. But maybe I'm the one who wants privacy.

These people hold up a mirror, and I pull back and shiver.

The next day I cry, and I'm relieved. It's triggered by seeing two people from my group hugging in the middle of the hall as we do some prayer/gratitude exercise. Initially I'm really cynical about the exercise and have to be talked into doing it, but then I see them embracing in the middle of the hall and it is this, for some reason, that touches me deeply, for I see suffering and love in both of them, and in them I see the suffering and love of everyone. And I also see something primitive and primal and Christ-like that I have pushed away, because I am an atheist, but this image of man and woman, like mother and son – his chest, her head, the interchange of them – connects with some old story that resides deep in me, and some feeling bursts like an explosion from my chest. And I know that if the only aim of the week is to drop down into a feeling state, then I've achieved it.

This is serenity – I really think this is it. It's come not from silence, but from noise, from diving deep and getting dirty. This feeling of serenity seems vastly different from the other times. It's not the blank, clear feeling I get from meditation. It feels fuller, like it could gush out of me. Yet I also feel more vulnerable, tentative and raw. My skin is thinner. I walk around feeling like every nerve is exposed, but in a good way.

When I return home, I slow things right down, and spend a lot of time outside. I can't be around certain people any more – people who are cynical or mean. I get up for the sunrise and take it all in with an almost tearful gratitude. I notice dust motes and watch them fall.

The feeling lasts for a long time, weeks and weeks. What a strange spell this is. It's continual ecstasy rolling at my feet. It's unlike anything I've experienced – but in it, there is no wanting (only wanting this feeling to stay forever). I don't need anything – everything I need I already have. The divine is within me and all others, I know that now. Everything is whole, everything is good, everything is as it should be. Serenity Now.

n the West we've moved at speed from a religious to a secular, atheist society. The liberation from old religions – especially for women – is immense, but with liberation comes some loss. There are consequences to this abrupt shedding of our spiritual skins. We've lost an important figment of the collective. Worshipping as a community is one less thing that we do together, one less thing that binds us. We've also lost the spirituality that used to be woven into how we lived. I still remember a time when no shops were open on Sunday, there was fish on Fridays and regular churchgoing, and religious holidays and saints days observed. That was my childhood. Now all that's gone – where I live, anyway. That other age has evaporated, unmourned – did it even happen?

How are we doing God-type experiences in a secular world? What is our source of serenity, *the peace that the world cannot give*? Where do we turn and what do we do if we want to go inwards? It's no coincidence that the rise of mindfulness meditation has emerged as organised religion has receded.

Modern life has very few gaps in it for us to practise the kind of intentional introspection and seek the serenity once found in traditional religion. Now spirituality is untethered from religion and is a commodity like any other product. To find it you need time, privilege and capital. Pay $2000 to go on retreat, and meaning, spirituality and community will be sold to you. You'll feel great for a week, connected, cleansed and whole (elated, even), but it's about as practical and as healthy as losing weight in the *Biggest Loser* house; there's little possibility or means of integrating what you've learnt into your daily life.

On that last day on retreat in Bali, I looked around my fellow retreaters (who I loved so much at the time, then never saw again) and wondered: how many of their prayer beads and string bracelets would survive the journey home? How many totems and amulets would be shoved to the back of a drawer? At home there may be no community waiting, no place to visit to get that sense of higher meaning, no one willing to dive below the surface with you, and so you go back to that empty feeling, until you go online and book another retreat – and the cycle starts anew.

Back in 2005 when I was going to evangelical churches in Sydney, many of the young people I interviewed weren't so much interested in God as they were in community and boundaries (real, not virtual communities, and moral boundaries) – two of the things missing in modern life. They were living in an individualistic world of moral relativism and were casting around for something, anything, that bound them together and fenced them in. The young evangelicals (who did three- or four-year stretches at their churches until their virginity bored them, or they became jaded and moved on, or that particular framework of meaning no longer fitted them) were easy to mock, but I understood them. You can have too much freedom and too much choice. Finding, establishing and maintaining a spiritual practice that has elements of introspection, whether it be prayer or meditation – I'm not saying it will lead to permanent happiness, but it can lead to serenity. And maybe that's the only pure, reliable form of happiness, because it is not reliant on external things: a hot boyfriend, a great job, lots of money in the bank. Those things come and go.

One of the awesome results of being unhooked from an ancestral religious tradition is that we are now free, perhaps freer than ever before, to forge our own path. It's one of the great miracles of our age that I could find myself deep in the Sri Lankan jungle in some moist mud hut, wrapped in a sheet while a quart of oil dripped from the ceiling (*drip-drip-drip-drip*) onto my third eye, following some ancient Ayurvedic healing tradition. Or practise Sufi meditation on the roof of a temple in Bali, or cloister myself with Benedictine monks in the wheat fields of Western Australia. What a time to be alive!

But, as I found, you can try all these spiritual traditions in the search for serenity, but trying ain't the same as living it. You cannot thin-slice faith. The serenity won't last.

Serenity is needed more than ever, but is harder to find. It's no surprise one of the hottest consumer products is noise-cancelling headphones. The noise isn't going to stop, so we have to create a product that prevents us from hearing – which seems the wrong way round. Blocking things rather than opening up: masking, masking, masking – it's all we can do. But we live in a world that conspires against stillness and silence, the very things needed to drop us down and into a state of serenity.

The neoliberal agenda is not conducive to serenity: closing down the public libraries, getting us all onto private, user-pays health care, selling off housing stock to cashed-up foreign investors, starving public schools of money, raping the environment for private profit, weakening unions, removing penalty rates ... the list goes on. But no matter! In your contract job, which might go for six weeks or might get extended (a job that doesn't provide any protections such as sick leave or holiday pay), there's this great initiative. They have mindfulness classes at lunchtime that are really great for chilling everyone out, because everyone's really stressed at the moment ... because no one knows if their contracts are going to be renewed. This time round mindfulness and self-care have been given to us by the market so we can comfort and lull ourselves into a non-panicked space, where we can soothe ourselves that these rough seas we ride on will not be the death of us.

In his book *Evil Paradises*, Mike Davis talks about the dreamworlds of neoliberalism, the physical spaces that money and globalisation have thrown up. The book describes these 'phantasmagoric but real places – alternate realities being constructed as "utopias" in a capitalist era unfettered by unions and state regulation'. Canggu in Bali is one of those places. I went there last year. Yoga studios and coffee shops have sprung up in the small seaside community seemingly overnight. Locals said that in the last two or three years there had been a massive wellness-related building boom. It looked like the good life, it looked like a *well* life; Melbourne-style flat whites at a cafe called Little Flinders in the morning after your ninety-minute vinyasa class in the soaring, cathedral-like bamboo yoga shala, followed by a swim or a surf, then an organic juice.

But some of the locals I met weren't so pleased. The boom was so intense that that corner of Bali was expected to run out of water within five years. There had been no plans made for this possibility. The spectre of environmental collapse was all around. Cranes crowded the skyline along the beach; Westerners on mopeds with surfboard racks clogged the unpaved roads to the beach and yoga studios. Huge concrete hotels were being built, with construction work going seven days a week and into the night. We want wellness and we want it now! I pondered the madness of this: in our search for inner peace and serenity we are prepared to rip up the planet. And, as a consumer of this stuff, I was a part of the problem.

In this age of anxiety, no wonder wellness holds such allure. In the yoga studio you can retreat from the harsh world out there and focus on your own body – its strengths and its limitations. In the wellness industry the personal isn't political any more, it is just purely personal. It's a different sort of border control. It is the borders that stop at your skin. In the name of wellness, you can hide from all the horror in plain sight, disguise your stasis with movement on the floor. The meditation in the morning will calm you down and keep you centred; the yoga class is not only a great workout but also has a spiritual lineage going back thousands of years that tethers you to something deeper than the weightless, flowing data that enthrals us and chains us to our smart phones. The organic food and detoxes and juices are a way of signalling that even though the world is going to shit, you still have control over what you put into your body. Control when there is no control over anything else, when 'all that is solid melts into air'.

When the great ideological and global projects appear to fail, there is still the Project of Self. The world is sick; the natural environment is dying – coral turning white before our eyes, like a cancer metastasising too fast to treat. No wonder we seek to bury ourselves in wholefoods, wellness memes, yoga classes and meditation apps.

The wellness industry can help us get clean and lean and serene, but the things that we have lost – the collective and the community, compassion and generosity – these are part of the great project too. There's no point reaching the beautiful summit, where we look good, feel great and are at peace, if we're there alone. Somewhere along the line when we were talking about the struggle, it turned lethally inwards. We could only see ourselves; others ceased to exist. The narcissism and solipsism were total. We became the women walking around their clotheslines, around and around in circles, treading the same ground until it wore a groove that we couldn't get out of, obsessed to the point of mania with our own bodies, our individual glow.

The time has come to look up, to step out of this worn path. The struggle has to mean something else now, something involving others, lifting others up. I sense something changing. There is a whiff of a return to the spirit of collectivism. You see it in the women's marches and the protests around Trump's Muslim ban. We've had years of looking after ourselves. Now it's time to look after each other.

AFTER

Over the past twelve years I've tried lots and lots of the products and offerings from the wellness industry. Some things have worked, some have been snake oil, and some were neutral – as in, they were fine, but didn't effect much real or lasting change.

Detoxes are fascinating and gruelling but can be risky. Ultimately they are seeking to do what the body already does with its lungs and kidneys and liver – filter out 'toxins'. You can do a detox and see some amazing results (like I did) – but with any rapid weight loss, it has been scientifically proven again and again that the weight will return (as it did with me).

I tried yoga for years without much improvement until I started doing it every day – then I saw many positive changes in my body, including improved strength and muscle tone, a 'glow' that comes with regular exercise, and increased stamina and energy. But once I moved away from the studio, when I started travelling a lot, the practice fell away. My body immediately started to feel locked up and stiff again. As I've spent long hours crunched over writing this book in a country town far from my favourite yoga studios, I've developed a real nostalgia for Namaste Dudes and the feeling I had after a great session.

Of course, other exercise regimes can deliver great benefits, but yoga gets you in touch with the more subtle energy systems in your body. And as for the nuggets of truth – in this secular world (where in the last couple of years, politically, environmentally and socially we appear to be in a state of decline, not progress), sometimes we need some wisdom or moral teaching, even if it is delivered when we are on our knees, in our ath-leisure gear, sweating in a semi-darkened studio. But it's a privilege to be able to practise every day – to be close to a good studio and have the time and money to do it. It is increasingly becoming a rich person's practice. A casual class at my studio of choice (not a fancy studio) is around twenty-seven dollars.

If you do one thing from this book, I would recommend shooting for serenity. Nothing has stuck for me quite like Vedic meditation. I do it most days. It works. But every teacher and every experience has been really helpful. Aruna was a revelation, turning my mind to a new way of being – that is, being in the present moment is the only thing that matters. *The past is a graveyard, the future doesn't exist.* It made me stand at one remove from my mind and notice how it races ahead, freaking me out. Mindfulness has been corrupted by market forces, but that doesn't diminish its fundamental value and purpose, which is to create a pocket of stillness and calm in your body and mind. We are in the age of distraction – we need an antidote.

But as I found time and time again, getting the knowledge is only the start. Next you have to apply it. Then you have to integrate it. Then you have to build it into your daily routine. Otherwise the improvements are temporary, and you go back to the easy comforts, the numbness or anxiety, the stiff, aching body. It's ongoing. Each day we must make ourselves anew.

ACKNOWLEDGEMENTS

My editor, Jo Rosenberg, plus Kelly Fagan and Emma Schwarcz, and my agent, Pippa Masson.

Friends who read bits and helped me tease out and refine ideas: Erik Jensen, Jemma Birrell, Jackie Dent, Jenny Valentish, Lee Glendinning, Tom Dobson, Gareth Hutchens, Adam Brereton, Julia Leigh, Bridie Jabour, Michael Safi, Zoe Beech Coyle, Joh Leggatt and Sharon Verghis.

My editors at *Guardian Australia*: Emily Wilson, Will Woodward and Gabrielle Jackson

My editors at *Sunday Life*: Danielle Teutsch (who started this whole ball rolling with the fast), Kate Cox and Pat Ingram.

My generous interview subjects: Adam Whiting, Phoebe Loomes, Matt Ringrose, Samved Dass and Alima Cameron.

My parents: Jim and Mary Delaney, and the Bundanon Trust for a residency, which was both peaceful and productive.

Plus – all those wonderful, curious, excellent and eccentric people I met along the wellness way. From all of you I learnt something.

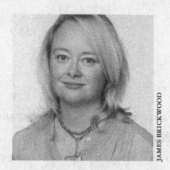

JAMES BRICKWOOD

Brigid Delaney is the author of *Wellmania*, *This Restless Life*, *Wild Things* and a book explaining Stoic philosophy – *Reasons Not to Worry*. She has worked as a columnist and journalist for *Guardian Australia*, and is currently a speechwriter for a federal minister.